How Did Researchers Reduce Hypertension?

Adam Kuzdraliński, PhD DSc.

DEDICATION

Dedicated to my daughter, wife, parents, sisters and to all who believe that it's never too late to make your dreams come true.

CONTENTS

ACKNOWLEDGMENTS

Thank you to everyone who contributed to the fact that I now have additional time to write; otherwise, this book would not have been written at all.

INTRODUCTION

There are numerous books on the market that discuss how to manage hypertension, but I get the impression that a lot of them publish titles based on hunches, or even the beliefs of their authors. Meanwhile, in the scientific literature there is no lack of successful experiments in which reductions in blood pressure have been achieved, frequently also using non-medication treatments. The idea here is absolutely not to discourage readers from medicines, because very often they are absolutely necessary, but rather to demonstrate that dietary, lifestyle, supplement, and even yoga-related elements are also studied in scientific laboratories. Such experiments frequently produce a specific response to the question of whether a given approach worked or did not work on a particular set of individuals and, consequently, if there is a likelihood that it will also work on another group that was not included in the study.

The scientific studies from the past ten years that have been published in the well-known scientific database PubMed Central® (PMC), a free full-text collection of biomedical and life sciences journal literature, have been taken into consideration in this book. I chose the last 10 years to reduce the number of papers to be examined; otherwise, I might not have been able to finish this book in any respectable amount of time. Additionally, I restricted my search exclusively to clinical trials to ensure that the articles I examined were of top quality in terms of methodology. It's not that other publications are bad in quality, but in the case of clinical trials, quality is determined by the framework that must be fulfilled for an experiment to be labeled with such a caption. One of the many requirements that an experiment bearing the label "clinical trial" must fulfill is that it must either have a power analysis (that is, an answer to the question of whether the analyzed group of patients is sufficient to obtain representative conclusions) or that it must have properly planned study groups, one of which is the control group to which the intervention group is compared).

In this book, I have included 168 publications (clinical studies) on hypertension, the majority of which describe interventions on bigger or smaller groups of participants, mostly hypertensive persons. When these publications were analyzed, it became clear that it would be best to divide the book into sections based on the type of intervention, such as dietary interventions, supplementations, physical activity interventions, and other experiments that are challenging to fit into the aforementioned categories. In addition, in describing additional information related to the subject of the intervention, I cited 114 other publications.

The papers studied frequently differed significantly from one another in methodology and results presentation, so I made some compromises to avoid eliminating too many of them. Some readers may view these compromises as oversimplifications, while others will likely find them to be beneficial. What do I mean by that? I made the decision to refer only to systolic blood pressure (SBP), which is, the pressure exerted by the blood on the arterial walls when the heart beats. Another issue was the variety of methods used to measure blood pressure, from daytime blood pressure measurements taken in several repetitions, to nighttime, all-day, post-exercise, sedentary and other measurements. Although I tried to compare primarily daily blood pressure measurements, this wasn't always possible. Where it was not possible, I usually wrote how the result was obtained. It was also not always possible to obtain an exact result because the publication's authors displayed the outcome as a graph, in which case I generated a reading based on the graphs. The method I used to determine blood pressure decrease was the difference in blood pressure in the study group after the intervention minus the difference in blood pressure before the intervention. From this, I subtracted the difference in blood pressure that occurred in the control group (if such a difference occurred or if the blood pressure of the control group after the intervention was given). I didn't always have to count it because many publications' authors just stated the number.

In analyzing the methodologies of the publications, I decided that the limit for describing the methodology for the selected publication in detail would be a blood pressure reduction of 7 mm Hg or more on average. I outlined the methods used in articles that resulted in a statistically significant drop in blood pressure, but less than 7 mm Hg. As the material in the abstract was frequently insufficient to allow for a useful description of the methodology, only those papers that were available in full in English were included in the analysis.

I have added images (that I created myself) in the frames where I describe the interventions' methodologies so that readers may quickly see the interventions' most successful approaches and their results. Additionally, I made the decision to include emoticons to show the intervention's effectiveness. I made the assumption that one emoticon would represent a drop in blood pressure of 7 to 10 mm Hg, two would represent a drop of 10.1 to 14 mm Hg, and three would represent a drop of more than 14 mm Hg.
I think the majority of readers will find this book to be very helpful, whether they are experts in the field or just have high blood pressure

or are concerned about developing hypertension.

I do want readers to understand that this book is not a compilation of miraculous treatments for hypertension. Here, I'm referring to the efficacy of the presented methods. Please keep in mind that the intervention chosen has shown to be successful in a particular group of people who share selected characteristics. The clearest illustration of this is an analysis of multiple studies that describe the chosen type of intervention and found that in some groups of people there was no effect, in others there was a so-so effect, and in others there was a substantial drop in blood pressure. Therefore, think of the stated interventions as ones that increase your chances of reducing your blood pressure, but are by no means a certainty. Furthermore, regularity, which is sometimes neglected, has a significant impact on achieving specific outcomes. It is also important to keep in mind that a significant percentage of individuals in the populations, where the chosen intervention produced very positive results, also included individuals for whom the selected strategy had no noticeable impact.

Safety concerns rank among the most crucial topics. Even the simplest actions can be harmful, such as when you are taking blood pressure-lowering medications or other medications used in the treatment of chronic diseases. It's possible that the medication you're taking and the intervention plan outlined in this book will cause your blood pressure to drop too low. Additionally, drug-interfering compounds are frequently found in plants and supplements. Therefore, whenever you plan an intervention, I advise visiting a medical or nutritional specialist. Never disregard medical advice from your doctor or another qualified health provider because of anything you read in this book. Any changes that could have an impact on your treatment or care plan should always be discussed with your doctor or other healthcare provider.

Not all of the publications that were discussed were based on interventions that took several weeks or months. I sometimes mentioned one-time interventions that had results that I thought would be interesting to the reader. In some of the publications studied, the findings were based on surveys, also included because, in my opinion, the results may be useful to readers. However, I do not compare them to classic interventions in the chapter summaries and in the summary at the end of the book.

PART 1. NUTRITION

1.1 DIET

I compiled this section of the book based on 40 research studies that were submitted to PubMed Central® (PMC), a free full-text archive of biomedical and life sciences journal literature. The effects of the following dietary modifications on blood pressure have been studied:

- Blueberries
- Dairy products
- DASH (Dietary Approaches to Stop Hypertension)
- Dietary nitrate
- East Asian diet
- Gazpacho
- Japanese diet
- Low-fat diet
- Miso soup
- Oat bran
- Olive oil
- Salt
- Protein intake
- Beet
- Seafood
- Spirulina sauce
- Tomato juice

It is significant to note that this section does not cover dietary supplements, which are explored separately in Part 1.2.

The aforementioned interventions that have been shown to be effective against hypertension are presented in Figure 1. It's interesting that practically all of the research seemed to lower blood pressure. Studies were conducted for several of the interventions where the effect was not achieved as in the other trials (usually in cases where there was more than one study). For instance, 11 studies found the DASH diet to be effective, whereas the remaining three found no benefit.

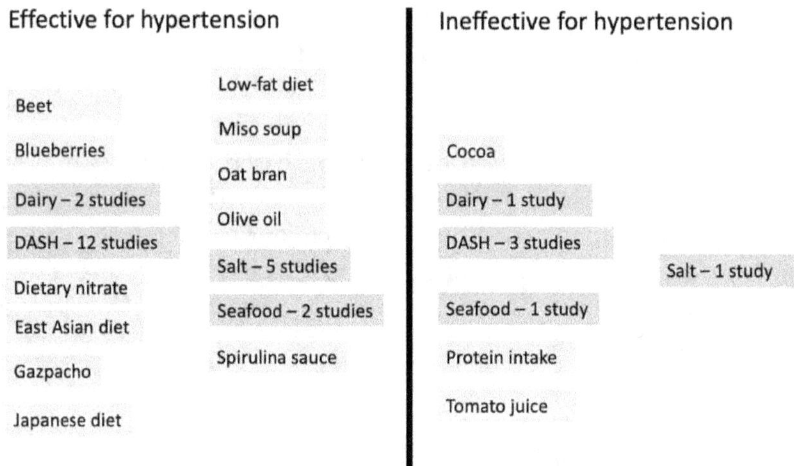

Figure 1. A comparison of types of interventions in relation to effects achieved, or not, against hypertension. Interventions are not ordered according to the effect obtained.

Only the dietary changes that have been proven to reduce blood pressure are included below. Therefore, studies on protein intake, tomato juice, and cocoa will not be discussed.

1.1.1 Blueberries

I only found one blueberry research study conducted in the past ten years (Johnson et al. 2015). Blood pressure in pre- and stage 1-hypertension in postmenopausal women from the US was reduced by 7 mm Hg. The study group consisted of 37 women, and their average age was 58.5 years.

Blueberries - how was the intervention conducted?

After 8 weeks of daily administration of 22 g (0.78 oz) of freeze-dried blueberry powder, the effect mentioned above was achieved. According to the scientific paper, this serving size is equivalent to exactly 1 cup of fresh blueberries. 11 g (0.39 oz) of tifblue (*Vaccinium virgatum*) and 11 g (0.39 oz) of rubel (*Vaccinium corymbosum*) made up the blueberry powder. Participants consumed half of the recommended daily intake (11 g = 0.39 oz) in the morning and the other half in the evening, at least 6 to 8 hours apart. Depending on their option, participants added Splenda or vanilla extract for flavor to the regimen.

What you should know

- *Vaccinium virgatum*, commonly known as smallflower blueberry or rabbit-eye blueberry is a native species to the Southeastern United States.
- *Vaccinium corymbosum* is one of the best-known blueberry species native to North America.
- One cup of berries contains 24% of the recommended daily intake of vitamin C for an adult.

- According to a very large scientific study, eating blueberries can considerably reduce the risk of developing type 2 diabetes (Muraki et al., 2013).
- Consuming blueberries might lead to slower rates of cognitive deterioration (Devore et al. 2012).
- Blueberries might lower blood sugar levels in people with diabetes and for this reason, be careful when consuming them along with medications that lower blood sugar.
- Salicylates, which can trigger allergies such as gastrointestinal problems, headaches, and rashes, can be found in blueberries in amounts as high as 27 mg per 100 g. Salicylic acid is a common aspirin.

References

1. Devore, E. E., Kang, J. H., Breteler, M. M., & Grodstein, F. (2012). Dietary intakes of berries and flavonoids in relation to cognitive decline. Annals of neurology, 72(1), 135-143.
2. Johnson, S. A., Figueroa, A., Navaei, N., Wong, A., Kalfon, R., Ormsbee, L. T., ... & Arjmandi, B. H. (2015). Daily blueberry consumption improves blood pressure and arterial stiffness in postmenopausal women with pre- and stage 1-hypertension: a randomized, double-blind, placebo-controlled clinical trial. Journal of the Academy of Nutrition and Dietetics, 115(3), 369-377.
3. Muraki, I., Imamura, F., Manson, J. E., Hu, F. B., Willett, W. C., van Dam, R. M., & Sun, Q. (2013). Fruit consumption and risk of type 2 diabetes: results from three prospective longitudinal cohort studies. Bmj, 347.

1.1.2 Dairy products

Three publications describe modifying one's diet by including conventional dairy products, whey protein, or calcium caseinate (Drouin-Chartier et al. 2014, Fekete et al. 2016, Maki et al. 2013). These results of these interventions can be regarded as being inconclusive. Only certain measurement types showed a blood pressure-lowering effect, and more frequently than not, there was no statistically significant effect. I will not go into detail about the approach or length of these interventions because the results are far from satisfactory.

References

1. Drouin-Chartier, J. P., Gigleux, I., Tremblay, A. J., Poirier, L., Lamarche, B., & Couture, P. (2014). Impact of dairy consumption on essential hypertension: a clinical study. Nutrition journal, 13(1), 1-9.
2. Fekete, A. A., Giromini, C., Chatzidiakou, Y., Givens, D. I., & Lovegrove, J. A. (2016). Whey protein lowers blood pressure and improves endothelial function and lipid biomarkers in adults with prehypertension and mild hypertension: results from the chronic Whey2Go randomized controlled trial. The American journal of clinical nutrition, 104(6), 1534-1544.
3. Maki, K. C., Rains, T. M., Schild, A. L., Dicklin, M. R., Park, K. M., Lawless, A. L., & Kelley, K. M. (2013). Effects of low-fat dairy intake on blood pressure, endothelial function, and lipoprotein lipids in subjects with prehypertension or stage 1 hypertension. Vascular health and risk management, 9, 369.

1.1.3 DASH diet

This type of intervention for hypertensive individuals is very popular in scientific papers. No wonder, since the DASH diet (Dietary Approaches to Stop Hypertension) was created to prevent and control hypertension. It seems like nothing new, but there are interesting findings from the 15 scientific studies analyzed (Azadbakht et al. 2016, Chen et al. 2012, Chiu et al. 2016, Couch et al. 2021, Epstein et al. 2012, Hummel et al. 2012, Kawamura et al. 2016, Kucharska et al. 2018, Lima et al. 2013, Paula et al. 2015, Saneei et al. 2013, Steinberg et al. 2019, Umemoto et al. 2020, Whitt-Glover et al. 2013, Wright et al. 2021).

Many of these papers' findings can be deemed to have outstanding results. A systolic blood pressure drop of more than 10 mm Hg was reported in as many as six articles. It is important to note that of these six articles, researchers used the DASH diet in five of them, either modified or in conjunction with another strategy. Four articles, however, failed to find an effect despite the fact that these treatments were linked to participant education.

I have compiled the results of these 15 experiments into a single graphic (Figure 2).

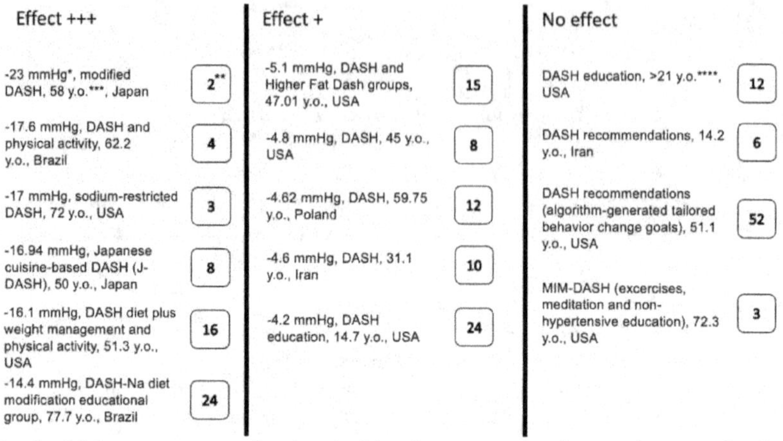

Effect +++		Effect +		No effect	
-23 mmHg*, modified DASH, 58 y.o.***, Japan	2**	-5.1 mmHg, DASH and Higher Fat Dash groups, 47.01 y.o., USA	15	DASH education, >21 y.o.****, USA	12
-17.6 mmHg, DASH and physical activity, 62.2 y.o., Brazil	4	-4.8 mmHg, DASH, 45 y.o., USA	8	DASH recommendations, 14.2 y.o., Iran	6
-17 mmHg, sodium-restricted DASH, 72 y.o., USA	3	-4.62 mmHg, DASH, 59.75 y.o., Poland	12	DASH recommendations (algorithm-generated tailored behavior change goals), 51.1 y.o., USA	52
-16.94 mmHg, Japanese cuisine-based DASH (J-DASH), 50 y.o., Japan	8	-4.6 mmHg, DASH, 31.1 y.o., Iran	10		
-16.1 mmHg, DASH diet plus weight management and physical activity, 51.3 y.o., USA	16	-4.2 mmHg, DASH education, 14.7 y.o., USA	24	MIM-DASH (excercises, meditation and non-hypertensive education), 72.3 y.o., USA	3
-14.4 mmHg, DASH-Na diet modification educational group, 77.7 y.o., Brazil	24				

* - the highest average reduction in blood pressure (understood as a reduction in systolic blood pressure) achieved by any of the measurement methods (daytime, nighttime, 24-hour, clinical, office, etc.)

** - number of weeks of dietary intervention

*** - average age of the study participants

**** - the average age of the participants was not given, only the age from which they were qualified for the experiment

Figure 2. Comparison of 15 studies where the DASH diet was used as the intervention.

DASH diet - how was the intervention conducted?

The American Heart Association recommends the commonly used dietary strategy known as DASH (Dietary Approaches to Stop Hypertension). The Japanese Guidelines for the Management of Hypertension also prescribe it, although due to significant cultural differences, the DASH diet is challenging for Japanese individuals to adhere to. Kawamura et al. (2016) examined the outcomes of an intervention using a modified DASH diet. They had the greatest outcomes for the DASH diet of the publications I examined. The DASH-JUMP (DASH-Japan Ube Modified Diet Program) diet modification they created had the same nutrient makeup as the original DASH diet.

The DASH-JUMP meals were designed with 2 calorie levels in mind (1650 for women and 1820 for men each day). This is less than the original DASH diet, which recommended an intake of 2100 kcal per day. DASH-JUMP had greater protein and carbs but less total fat and saturated fatty acids. Numerous fruits, veggies, and low-fat dairy products are present in DASH-JUMP. No matter the daily caloric intake, each variant's meals (1650 and 1820 kcal) contained approximately 8 g (0.28 oz) of salt per day.

Sample meals of the DASH-JUMP diet included in the described article:

- Breakfast
    - Tea rice gruel,
    - Food boiled and seasoned with tofu, Japanese radish and carrot,
    - Lotus root dumplings,
    - Low sodium soy sauce,
    - Citrus natsudaidai jelly.

- Lunch
    - Green tea-soba, a shredded omelet and laver, noodle soup,
    - Boiled greens with dressing of rape oil,
    - Food item formed by wrapping and twisting a tea cloth into the shape of a pumpkin.

- Dinner
    - Rice sprouts,
    - Rico soup containing spinach and turnip,
    - Pickled vegetables with red pepper and horse mackerel,
    - Mushrooms sautéed in butter,
    - Powdered green tea milk.

Paula et al. (2015) found that when the DASH diet and exercise were combined in 40 Brazilians with type 2 diabetes and hypertension, the blood pressure was significantly lowered.

Intervention characteristics:

- 25 to 30 kcal per kilogram of body weight,
- nutritional composition: 55% of calories comes from carbohydrates, 18% from proteins, and 27% from total fat,
- salt, fats, and sweets were discouraged;
- consumption of vegetables, low-fat dairy, whole grains, lean meats, nuts, seeds, and beans was promoted;
- participants were instructed to eat wholegrain bread and soy oil;

- physical activity: in addition to their regular activities, they should walk for at least 15 to 20 minutes per day, five days a week.

Sample diet for a person with type 2 diabetes, weighing 70 kg (154,32 lb) from the Paula et al. (2015) article:

- Breakfast
  - wholegrain bread (2 slices - 50 g = 1.76 oz),
  - mozzarella cheese (1 slice - 15 g = 0.53 oz),
  - skim milk (1 cup - 150 ml),
  - coffee (50 ml)
- Snack 1:
  - 1 fruit (100 g = 3.53 oz)
- Lunch
  - vegetable A (freely),
  - vegetable B   (3 tablespoons - 60 g = 2.12 oz),
  - rice or other (3 tablespoons - 60 g = 2.12 oz),
  - beans (1 small scoop - 60 g = 2.12 oz),
  - lean meat (1 medium piece - 90 g = 3.17 oz),
  - fruit (1 serving - 100 g = 3.53 oz)
- Snack 2
  - skimmed yogurt (1 cup - 120 g = 4.23 oz),
  - fruit (1 serving - 100 g = 3.53 oz)
- Dinner
  - vegetable A (freely),
  - vegetable B (3 tablespoons - 60 g = 2.12 oz),
  - rice or other (3 tablespoons - 60 g = 2.12 oz),
  - lean meat (1 medium piece - 90 g = 3.17 oz),
  - fruit (1 serving - 100 g = 3.53 oz)

Additionally, after adopting the DASH diet modification (DASH/SRD), where additional sodium restriction was implemented (1.15 g(0.04 oz) of sodium/2100 kcal/day), patients with heart failure saw excellent improvements. Sample diet from Hummel et al. (2012):

- Breakfast
  - oatmeal cooked (1 cup = 234 g = 8.25 oz),
  - margarine (1 pat),
  - almonds ¼ cup (30 g = 1.06 oz),

- brown sugar (18 g = 0.63 oz),
  - banana (1 = 70 g = 2.47 oz),
  - orange juice (4 ounces = ½ of cup),
  - skim milk (4 ounces = ½ of cup).
- Lunch
  - tossed romaine greens (120 g = 4.23 oz),
  - baked chicken breast (3.7 ounces = 110 g),
  - sliced cucumbers (5 slices = 76 g = 2.68 oz),
  - grapes (1 cup = 150 g = 5.29 oz),
  - almonds (¼ cup = 30 g = 1.06 oz),
  - diet Italian dressing (2 packets),
  - wheat roll (1 = 95 g = 3.35 oz),
  - straw/banana lite yogurt (6 ounces = ¾ of cup).
- Dinner
  - minestrone soup (150 g = 5.29 oz),
  - white roll (28 g = 0.99 oz),
  - roast turkey (100 g = 3.53 oz),
  - gravy (2 tablespoons = 43 g = 1.52 oz),
  - orzo pasta (150 g = 5.29 oz),
  - broccoli florets (1 cup = 164 g = 5.78 oz),
  - margarine (2 pats).
- Snack
  - skim milk (4 ounces = ½ of cup),
  - oat/honey bar (1 bar = 21 g = 0.74 oz),
  - orange (1).

Following this diet, people's average blood pressure decreased from 155 to 138 mm Hg after just 3 weeks.

A DASH diet modification called Japanese cuisine-based DASH (J-DASH) was tested on a group of 40 Japanese participants with normal-high blood pressure or stage 1 hypertension who had never taken antihypertensive medication prior to the experiment. Umemoto et al. (2020) reported very good outcomes. This diet is a variation of the DASH-JUMP diet that was previously discussed in this book. They were able to lower the average systolic blood pressure in several test groups by almost 17 mm Hg. Participants also received instruction on diet and healthy eating practices. It is significant to note that the J-DASH diet was lower in fat and saturated fatty acids than the original DASH diet. Participants could eat whatever they liked throughout the weekend, and liquids were not included in the regimen, so they could still drink coffee and alcohol. All participants were also required to consume 50 grams (1.76 oz) of commercial cereal (Calbee Frugra) during breakfast. The authors identified 2 study groups, one of which consumed only 1 meal per day on the J-DASH diet (the remaining meal was the participant's usual meal or choice) and the other consumed 2 meals per day on the J-DASH diet. Thus, as can be seen, part of the diet was consistent with the classic diet of the studied group. Although the article omitted the diet's specifics, it can be deduced that it was comparable to the previously mentioned DASH-JUMP diet.

In sedentary, overweight, and obese hypertensive individuals from the US, the DASH diet alone (DASH-A group) or in conjunction with behavioral weight management (DASH+WM group) for 14 weeks reduced blood pressure on average by up to 16.1 mm Hg from baseline (blood pressure prior to intervention) (Epstein et al. 2012). Importantly, the intervention included weekly 30-45 minute sessions with the research dietitian leading support and feedback (DASH-A and DASH-WM). The DASH-WM group meetings also included a psychologist. Calorie restrictions, behavior changes, and 30-45 minutes of aerobic exercise three times a week were additionally advised. Although there are no specific suggestions or a sample diet in this article, there is a grading system that can be used to determine the overall advice given to the participants - 0.5 points were given for following the recommendation accurately, 1 point was given for eating more than the recommended amount, and 0 points were given for eating less:

- total grain: ≥ 7 servings/d (1), 5–6 servings/d (0.5), <5 servings/d (0),
- vegetables: ≥ 4 servings/d (1), 2-3 servings/d (0.5), <2 servings/d (0),
- fruits: ≥ 4 servings/d (1), 2-3 servings/d (0.5), <2 servings/d (0),
- dairy: ≥ 2 servings/d (1), 1 serving/d (0.5), <1 serving/d (0),
- meat, poultry, and fish: ≤ 2 servings/d (1), 3 servings/d (0.5), ≥ 4 servings/d (0),
- nuts, seeds, and dry beans: ≥ 4 servings/d (1), 2-3 servings/d (0.5), 2 servings/d (0),

- % kcal from fat: ≤27% (1), 28-29% (0.5), ≥30% (0),
- % kcal from saturated fat: ≤6% (1), 7-8% (0.5), ≥9% (0),
- sweets: ≤5 servings/wk (1), 6-7 servings/wk (0.5), ≥8 serving/wk (0),
- sodium: ≤2400 mg/d (1), 2400-3000 mg/d (0.5), >3000 mg/d (0).

It's important to note that the average drop in blood pressure in the DASH-A group was 11.2 mm Hg, whereas the average reduction in the DASH-WM group was 16.1 mm Hg. This means that adding more recommendations and physical activity increased the outcome by 44%.

The most recent study with the greatest impact on the DASH diet was published by Lima et al. (2013), who found that the Brazilian DASH diet educational group experienced an average blood pressure decrease of 14.4 mm Hg. This study focused on the intervention of modifying the low-glycemic index Brazilian diet combined with the principles of the DASH-Na (DASH plus salt intake reduction) diet. Dietary advice was given to participants on a monthly basis, emphasizing foods with a low to moderate glycemic index (GI, 70) and encouraging a greater intake of fruits, vegetables, low-fat dairy products, beans, and cassava while discouraging a greater intake of salt, meat and meat products, and sugary beverages. The diet was high in potassium, magnesium, and fiber and low in refined grains, salt, sugar, and saturated and total fat.

Participants were asked to consume 5-6 meals per day:
- 2 servings of low-fat milk,
- 3 to 5 servings of fruit,
- 4-5 servings of vegetables,
- 1 serving of legumes,
- 5-9 servings of cereals, roots and tubers,
- 1-2 servings of meat, primarily fish.

Food groups included in the menu:
- Breakfast and snacks
  - Milk products: skim milk, cream cheese, white low-fat farmer's cheese and low-fat yogurt
  - Bread: wholegrain bread, French bread, oat (oat bran), maize or rice, maize couscous or preparation

of maize, cassava, whole grain or water cracker
- o Fruits : avocado, pineapple, acerola, banana, hog-plum, cashew, star fruit, guava, jackfruit, orange, lemon, apple, mango, papaya, passion fruit, watermelon, melon, pear, pitomba, sapodilla, tangerine, grape
- Lunch and dinner
  - o Cereals (every day): parboiled/coarse rice, rice with vinegar or other greens and pasta
  - o Beans (every day): bean and soy
  - o Green vegetables: cabbage leaf, lettuce and vinegar
  - o Others vegetables: carrots, cabbage, cassava, cucumber, eggplant, gherkin, onion, okra, pepper, pumpkin, tomato, sweet potato/potatoes and pod
  - o Meats, eggs and fish: lean meat, beef liver, bovine viscera (tripe/sweetbreads), eggs (egg white), fish, skinless chicken, sardine, tuna, shrimp and mussels
  - o Desserts: fruits, jellied fruit and jam
  - o Soups: vegetables and beans without rice or pasta
- Oils: olive oil and soybean oil
- Spices: garlic, bay leaf, chive, coriander, oregano, parsley leaf and pepper

What you should know
- The DASH diet recommends the frequent consumption of:
  - o fruits (4-5 servings per day),
  - o vegetables (4-5 servings per day),
  - o whole grains (6-8 servings per day),
  - o low-fat or fat-free dairy products (2-3 servings per day),
  - o meats, poultry and fish (3-4 one-ounce servings or less per day),
  - o nuts, seeds and legumes (3-5 one-ounce servings or less per day),
  - o vegetable oils (2-3 servings a day).
- The DASH diet recommends avoiding:
  - o sugary beverages,
  - o full-fat dairy products,
  - o sweets,

- o chips,
- o cookies,
- o pastries,
- o snacks,
- o salt consumption,
- o fatty meats.
- The DASH diet may also lower LDL cholesterol levels, reduces blood uric acid in people with hyperuricemia, prevent the development of diabetes and even some kidney diseases (Harvard T.H. Chan School of Public Health, website).

References

1. Azadbakht, L., Izadi, V., Ehsani, S., & Esmaillzadeh, A. (2016). Effects of the dietary approaches to stop hypertension (DASH) eating plan on the metabolic side effects of corticosteroid medications. Journal of the American College of Nutrition, 35(4), 285-290.

2. Chen, Q., Turban, S., Miller, E. R., & Appel, L. J. (2012). The effects of dietary patterns on plasma renin activity: results from the Dietary Approaches to Stop Hypertension trial. Journal of human hypertension, 26(11), 664-669.

3. Chiu, S., Bergeron, N., Williams, P. T., Bray, G. A., Sutherland, B., & Krauss, R. M. (2016). Comparison of the DASH (Dietary Approaches to Stop Hypertension) diet and a higher-fat DASH diet on blood pressure and lipids and lipoproteins: a randomized controlled trial–3. The American journal of clinical nutrition, 103(2), 341-347.

4. Couch, S. C., Saelens, B. E., Khoury, P. R., Dart, K. B., Hinn, K., Mitsnefes, M. M., ... & Urbina, E. M. (2021). Dietary approaches to stop hypertension dietary intervention improves blood pressure and vascular health in youth with elevated blood pressure. Hypertension, 77(1), 241-251.

5. Epstein, D. E., Sherwood, A., Smith, P. J., Craighead, L., Caccia, C., Lin, P. H., ... & Blumenthal, J. A. (2012). Determinants and consequences of adherence to the dietary approaches to stop hypertension diet in African-American and white adults with high blood pressure: results from the ENCORE trial. Journal of the Academy of Nutrition and Dietetics, 112(11), 1763-1773.

6. Harvard T.H. Chan School of Public Health, Diet Review: DASH, The Nutrition Source. (2018, January 16). The Nutrition Source. https://www.hsph.harvard.edu/nutritionsource/healthy-weight/diet-reviews/dash-diet/

7. Hummel, S. L., Seymour, E. M., Brook, R. D., Kolias, T. J., Sheth, S. S., Rosenblum, H. R., ... & Weder, A. B. (2012). Low-sodium dietary approaches to stop hypertension diet reduces blood pressure, arterial stiffness, and oxidative stress in hypertensive heart failure with preserved ejection fraction. Hypertension, 60(5), 1200-1206.

8. Kawamura, A., Kajiya, K., Kishi, H., Inagaki, J., Mitarai, M., Oda, H., ... & Kobayashi, S. (2016). Effects of the DASH-JUMP dietary intervention in Japanese participants with high-normal blood pressure and stage 1 hypertension: an open-label single-arm trial. Hypertension Research, 39(11), 777-785.

9. Kucharska, A., Gajewska, D., Kiedrowski, M., Sińska, B., Juszczyk, G., Czerw, A., ... & Niegowska, J. (2018). The impact of individualised nutritional therapy according to DASH diet on blood pressure, body mass, and selected biochemical parameters in overweight/obese patients with primary arterial hypertension: a prospective randomised study. Kardiologia Polska (Polish Heart Journal), 76(1), 158-165.

10. Lima, S. T. R. M., de Souza, B. D. S. N., França, A. K. T., Salgado Filho, N., & Sichieri, R. (2013). Dietary approach to hypertension based on low glycaemic index and principles of DASH (Dietary Approaches to Stop Hypertension): a randomised trial in a primary care service. British journal of nutrition, 110(8), 1472-1479.

11. Paula, T. P., Viana, L. V., Neto, A. T., Leitao, C. B., Gross, J. L., & Azevedo, M. J. (2015). Effects of the DASH diet and walking on blood pressure in patients with type 2 diabetes and uncontrolled hypertension: a randomized controlled trial. The Journal of Clinical Hypertension, 17(11), 895-901.

12. Saneei, P., Hashemipour, M., Kelishadi, R., Rajaei, S., & Esmaillzadeh, A. (2013). Effects of recommendations to follow the Dietary Approaches to Stop Hypertension (DASH) diet v. usual dietary advice on childhood metabolic syndrome: a randomised cross-over clinical trial. British Journal of Nutrition, 110(12), 2250-2259.

13. Steinberg, D., Kay, M., Burroughs, J., Svetkey, L. P., & Bennett, G. G. (2019). The effect of a digital behavioral weight loss intervention on adherence to the dietary approaches to stop hypertension (DASH) dietary pattern in medically vulnerable primary care patients: results from a randomized controlled trial. Journal of the Academy of Nutrition and Dietetics, 119(4), 574-584.

14. Umemoto, S., Onaka, U., Kawano, R., Kawamura, A., Motoi, S., Honda, N., ... & J-DASH Diet Study Group. (2020). Effects of a Japanese cuisine-based antihypertensive diet and fish oil on blood pressure and its variability in participants with untreated normal high blood pressure or stage I hypertension: a feasibility randomized controlled study. Journal of Atherosclerosis and Thrombosis, 57802.

15. Whitt-Glover, M. C., Hunter, J. C., Foy, C. G., Quandt, S. A., Vitolins, M. Z., Leng, I., ... & Bertoni, A. G. (2013). Translating the Dietary Approaches to Stop Hypertension (DASH) diet for use in underresourced, urban African American communities, 2010.

16. Wright, K. D., Klatt, M. D., Adams, I. R., Nguyen, C. M., Mion, L. C., Tan, A., ... & Scharre, D. W. (2021). Mindfulness in motion and dietary approaches to stop hypertension (DASH) in hypertensive African Americans. Journal of the American Geriatrics Society, 69(3), 773-778.

1.1.4 Dietary nitrate

According to Kerley et al. (2018), participants with known or suspected uncontrolled hypertension saw an 8 mm Hg reduction in blood pressure on average after 7 days of consuming nitrate-rich beetroot juice (nitrate content: 7.5 mmol per 250 ml). The authors claim that this level of nitrate is consistent with a diet high in vegetables.

Dietary nitrate - how was the intervention conducted?

Each morning at around 9:00 am, participants drank 140 ml of nitrate-rich beetroot juice. All the participants received information on lifestyle choices that may prevent the absorption of nitrates, including those related to diet, alcohol, cigarettes, exercise, and medication use, as well as advice not to use mouthwash or antibiotics for the same reason.

What know should you

- Dietary nitrate can be found in green leafy vegetables and root vegetables including spinach, mustard greens, arugula, kale, Swiss chard, lettuce, beets, radishes, turnips, watercress, etc.
- Nitrate supplementation can, in some circumstances, enhance exercise tolerance and performance (Jones, 2014).
- Nitrates are naturally present in food and the human body. Additionally, nitrates are added to processed foods to lengthen their shelf lives. The high-temperature cooking of nitrates might result in the formation of harmful nitrosamines. However, compared to cooking meat, cooking vegetables is less likely to produce nitrosamines. Other bioactive substances, such as vitamin C, can inhibit the

formation of nitrosamines when nitrate is consumed as part of a regular diet that includes vegetables.

- The creation of nitrosamines is typically significantly inhibited by antioxidants from fruits and vegetables; if the amount of antioxidants is two times that of nitrates, the conversion process to nitrosamines is completely stopped (Karwowska and Kononiuk, 2020).

References

1. Jones, A. M. (2014). Dietary nitrate supplementation and exercise performance. Sports medicine, 44(1), 35-45.
2. Karwowska, M., & Kononiuk, A. (2020). Nitrates/nitrites in food—Risk for nitrosative stress and benefits. Antioxidants, 9(3), 241.
3. Kerley, C. P., Dolan, E., James, P. E., & Cormican, L. (2018). Dietary nitrate lowers ambulatory blood pressure in treated, uncontrolled hypertension: a 7-d, double-blind, randomised, placebo-controlled, cross-over trial. British Journal of Nutrition, 119(6), 658-663.

1.1.5 East Asian mimicking diet

53 Korean adults with type 2 diabetes were investigated in the 12-week trial by Jin et al. (2021). The average blood pressure dropped by 1.9 mm Hg when the Mediterranean and DASH diets were combined, which resemble the typical East Asian diet. I will not go into detail about the authors' methods due to the modest effect.

References

1. Jin, S. M., Ahn, J., Park, J., Hur, K. Y., Kim, J. H., & Lee, M. K. (2021). East Asian diet-mimicking diet plan based on the Mediterranean diet and the Dietary Approaches to Stop Hypertension diet in adults with type 2 diabetes: A randomized controlled trial. Journal of diabetes investigation, 12(3), 357-364.

1.1.6 Gazpacho

A large study conducted by Medina-Remón et al. (2013) examined the potential effects of consuming gazpacho on 3962 volunteers from Spain. Surprisingly, both the group with a moderate intake (1–19 g/d) and the group with a high intake (>20 g/d) of gazpacho showed a decrease in blood pressure. The abundance of phytochemicals in gazpacho, according to the authors, helps to explain this. However, I also will not discuss the methods because the blood pressure reduction in this instance (by 2.6–2.8 mm Hg) was not sufficient.

References

1. Medina-Remón, A., Vallverdú-Queralt, A., Arranz, S., Ros, E., Martinez-Gonzalez, M. A., Sacanella, E., ... & Lamuela-Raventos, R. M. (2013). Gazpacho consumption is associated with lower blood pressure and reduced hypertension in a high cardiovascular risk cohort. Cross-sectional study of the PREDIMED trial. Nutrition, Metabolism and Cardiovascular Diseases, 23(10), 944-952.

1.1.7 Low fat diet

In their article published in 2016, Allison et al. present a very big experiment that included 48,835 individuals. This study sought to lower the risk of breast cancer by increasing vegetable, fruit, and grain consumption while keeping total fat intake at 20 percent of total energy. The researchers also took blood pressure readings, and they discovered that this diet marginally lowered it (by 0.66 mm Hg on average). I won't go into detail about the study's methodology due to the study's small effects.

References

1. Allison, M. A., Aragaki, A. K., Ray, R. M., Margolis, K. L., Beresford, S. A., Kuller, L., ... & Van Horn, L. (2016). A randomized trial of a low-fat diet intervention on blood pressure and hypertension: tertiary analysis of the WHI dietary modification trial. American journal of hypertension, 29(8), 959-968.

1.1.8 Miso soup

Traditional Japanese meal known as common miso is made with soybeans, malted rice, and salt. In an experiment, participants were given 16 g (0.56 oz) of avase miso (1.9 g salt = 0.07 oz) and 160 mL of hot water twice a day, according to Kondo et al. (2019). The authors of the study claim that while miso soup did not affect blood pressure during the day, it did lower it at night compared to the control group. Unfortunately, there are no numbers in the article to help evaluate the impact. It appears from the graphs that the effect was not especially notable.

References

1. Kondo, H., Sakuyama Tomari, H., Yamakawa, S., Kitagawa, M., Yamada, M., Itou, S., ... & Uehara, Y. (2019). Long-term intake of miso soup decreases nighttime blood pressure in subjects with high-normal blood pressure or stage I hypertension. Hypertension Research, 42(11), 1757-1767.

1.1.9 Oat bran

A study by Xue et al. (2021) examined 44 Chinese volunteers' blood pressure levels after they consumed oat bran for three months. As a result, there was a considerable decrease in blood pressure, with reductions of 10.4 mm Hg and 15.3 mm Hg.

Oat bran - how was the intervention conducted?

Each participant consumed one bag of oat bran (30 g = 1.06 oz) daily, either with breakfast or in between meals. Dietary advice was also part of the intervention, albeit everyone who took part—including those in the control group—received recommendations.

Dietary advice:

- <6 g per day of sodium (<0.21 oz),
- a low consumption of saturated fatty acids and cholesterol, such as animal viscera (sweetbreads/gizzards), cream products, and animal oil,
- 500 g per day (17.64 oz) of vegetables and fruits, such as lettuce, celery, apple, and banana,
- 50-70 g per week (1.76-2.47 oz) of nuts, such as almonds and peanuts,
- 400 g per week (14.11 oz) of fish,
- 200 ml per day of low-fat or skim dairy milk.

What you should know

- Oat bran contains significant amounts of beta-glucans, dietary fiber elements known to lower cholesterol levels and postprandial blood sugar levels (Rahar et al., 2011).
- A 12-week research study on ulcerative colitis patients discovered that consuming 60 grams of oat bran daily (2.12 oz) decreased reflux and stomach pain (Hallert et al., 2003).
- Oat bran is very rich in antioxidants, such as avenanthramides, which are found only in oats.
- Phytic acid, which can chelate metal ions, particularly zinc, calcium, and iron, is present in oat bran in amounts of about 6%. This means it's a good idea not to consume oat bran together with foods and supplements (Caballero, 2003).
- Bran contains fructan, one of several substances classified as a FODMAP (fermentable oligosaccharides, disaccharides, monosaccharides, and polyols). Eating a diet high in FODMAPs is believed to be linked to an increase in irritable bowel syndrome symptoms (Marsh et al 2016).

References

1. Caballero, B., Trugo, L. C., & Finglas, P. M. (2003). Encyclopedia of food sciences and nutrition. Academic.
2. Hallert, C., Björck, I., Nyman, M., Pousette, A., Gränno, C., & Svensson, H. (2003). Increasing fecal butyrate in ulcerative colitis patients by diet: controlled pilot study. Inflammatory bowel diseases, 9(2), 116-121.
3. Marsh, A., Eslick, E. M., & Eslick, G. D. (2016). Does a diet low in FODMAPs reduce symptoms associated with functional gastrointestinal disorders? A comprehensive systematic review and meta-analysis. European journal of nutrition, 55(3), 897-906.
4. Rahar, S., Swami, G., Nagpal, N., Nagpal, M. A., & Singh, G. S. (2011). Preparation, characterization, and biological properties of β-glucans. Journal of advanced pharmaceutical technology & research, 2(2), 94.
5. Xue, Y., Cui, L., Qi, J., Ojo, O., Du, X., Liu, Y., & Wang, X. (2021). The effect of dietary fiber (oat bran) supplement on blood pressure in patients

with essential hypertension: A randomized controlled trial. Nutrition, Metabolism and Cardiovascular Diseases, 31(8), 2458-2470.

1.1.10 Olive oil

In a study by Moreno-Luna et al. (2012), 24 women's blood pressure was monitored for 4 months as part of a Spanish experiment. The participants followed the same diet (Mediterranean-style diet), and one group received olive oil high in polyphenols while the other received olive oil low in polyphenols. Only the group that consumed olive oil high in polyphenols had a significant reduction in blood pressure, with an average drop of 7.91 mm Hg.

Olive oil - how was the intervention conducted?
The participants were instructed to take daily 60 ml of virgin olive oil containing 564 mg/kg polyphenols, which equaled around 30 milligrams of polyphenols.

What you should know
- The Mediterranean diet, which is recognized as one of the healthiest, includes olive oil as one of the main sources of fats.
- Refined, virgin, and extra-virgin olive oils are the three types that are commonly found. The greatest concentration of antioxidants that promote health is found in extra-virgin olive oil.
- Extra virgin olive oil polyphenols may lower the risk of cancer, heart disease, and cognitive dysfunction (Tressera-Rimbau et al., 2017).

- The consumption of raw olive oil in order to preserve its benefits is advised.
- Blood sugar may be lowered with olive oil (Schwingshackl et al. 2017).
- The predominant fatty acid in olive oil is oleic acid, which can make up to 70% of the total oil content, which reduces the synthesis of fatty acids and cholesterol (Gnoni et al., 2010).

References

1. Gnoni, G. V., Natali, F., Geelen, M. J., & Siculella, L. (2010). Oleic acid as an inhibitor of fatty acid and cholesterol synthesis. In Olives and olive oil in health and disease prevention (pp. 1365-1373). Academic Press.
2. Moreno-Luna, R., Muñoz-Hernandez, R., Miranda, M. L., Costa, A. F., Jimenez-Jimenez, L., Vallejo-Vaz, A. J., ... & Stiefel, P. (2012). Olive oil polyphenols decrease blood pressure and improve endothelial function in young women with mild hypertension. American journal of hypertension, 25(12), 1299-1304.
3. Schwingshackl, L., Lampousi, A. M., Portillo, M. P., Romaguera, D., Hoffmann, G., & Boeing, H. (2017). Olive oil in the prevention and management of type 2 diabetes mellitus: a systematic review and meta-analysis of cohort studies and intervention trials. Nutrition & diabetes, 7(4), e262-e262.
4. Tressera-Rimbau, A., Arranz, S., Eder, M., & Vallverdú-Queralt, A. (2017). Dietary polyphenols in the prevention of stroke. Oxidative medicine and cellular longevity, 2017.

1.1.11 Salt

Six studies describing experimental findings on the effects of salt intake on blood pressure were published during the time under consideration (de Brito-Ashurst et al. 2013, He et al. 2021, Hummel et al. 2012, Mu et al. 2020, Rahimdel et al. 2019, Yang et al. 2018). In five, a blood pressure-lowering impact was seen; the drop varied from 8 to 17 mm Hg. In one study, no effect was seen, but the intervention involved giving the participants access to an educational program (Rahimdel et al. 2019)

Salt - how was the intervention conducted?

Hummel et al. (2012) achieved the highest blood pressure reduction, which was previously mentioned in the DASH diet

---

section. In this study, participants were given the option to follow the DASH diet modified to include additional salt restriction (1.15 g(0.04 oz) of sodium/1,100 kcal/day). The DASH diet section includes a sample meal plan.

Mu et al. (2020) reduced blood pressure in Chinese participants by up to 16 mm Hg by using a salt alternative. This alternative had a sodium chloride content of 18%, a potassium content of 35%, and a calcium content of 10%. The participants were split into two groups, one of which did not use anti-hypertensive drugs at all or lowered their dosage during the experiment, and the other of which continued to do so. After 8 weeks, individuals who continued to take their medicine as prescribed experienced a decrease in blood pressure, but strangely, those who cut back or stopped taking their medication entirely did not experience an increase in blood pressure. The study participants were told to maintain their routines.

An intervention involving hands-on cooking classes and instructional sessions was carried out in Bangladeshi patients with chronic kidney disease and hypertension in the UK (de Brito-Ashurst et al. 2013). Two versions of their typical meals were prepared during the practical sessions; one followed the usual recipe, and the other had salt reduced by 50%. After six months, the study group had a drop in blood pressure (nighttime blood pressure) of up to an average of 12 mm Hg.

He et al. (2021) included 1698 Chinese people who had hypertension along with their families. In the first trial group, the intervention consisted of eating a diet containing 3 g of salt daily (0.11 oz), whereas in the second study group, the amount may reach 18 g (0.64 oz). The experiment lasted 14 days. Three groups—highly sodium-sensitive, moderately sodium-sensitive, and sodium-resistant—were created by the authors to divide the study participants. The low-sodium diet in the extremely sodium-sensitive group reduced blood pressure by an average of 13.7 mm Hg (in the moderately sodium-sensitive group: 4.9 mm Hg), whereas the high-sodium diet in the same group raised blood pressure by an average of 11.2 mm Hg. It's interesting to note that the authors found that among the participants, 18% responded with a large drop in blood pressure when dietary salt was reduced and a large increase when sodium intake was increased.

The effects of a low-sodium diet on Chinese hypertensive patients and those with isolated systolic hypertension (ISH) were studied by Yang et al. (2018). When the average of two office blood pressure readings is equal to or higher than 140 mm Hg and the average of the concurrently recorded diastolic blood pressure is less than 90 mm Hg, ISH is diagnosed. Only the ISH group experienced a mean blood pressure reduction of 8 mm Hg after six months of following a low-sodium diet. Unfortunately, there aren't enough intervention details in this study.

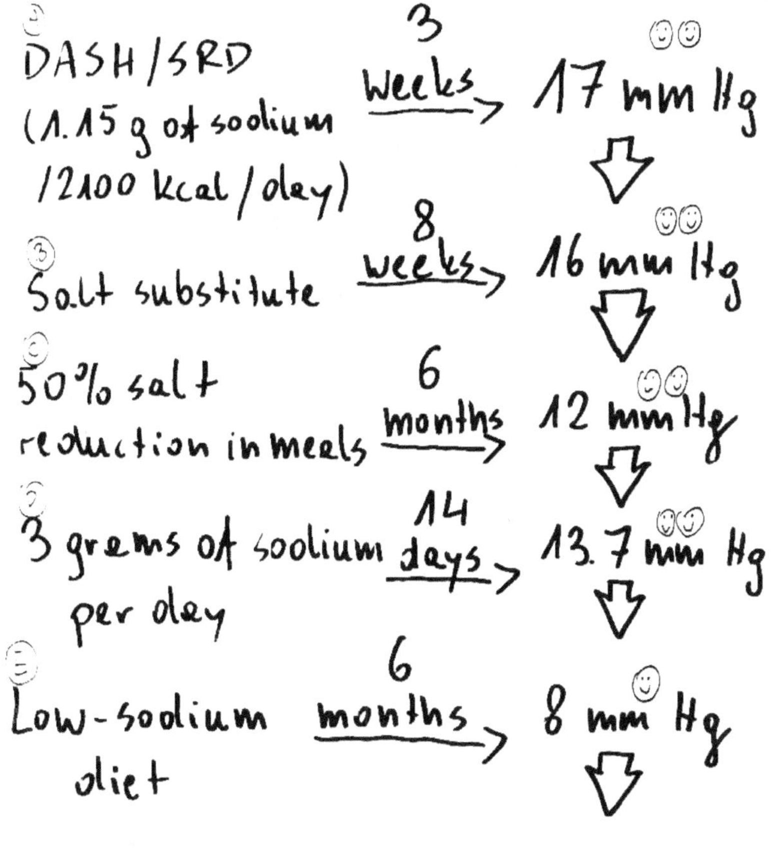

What you should know

- The WHO recommends reducing salt intake to less than 5 g/day per person, which is equal to about a teaspoon of salt (WHO, 2015).
- The daily sodium limit advised by the Dietary Guidelines for Americans is 2.3 grams (0.08 oz), or 5.8 grams of salt (0.21 oz) (CDC website).
- Reducing dietary salt intake by 3 grams per day (0.11 oz) is projected to reduce the annual number of new cases of Coronary Heart Disease by 60,000 to 120,000, stroke by 32,000 to 66,000, heart attack by 54,000 to 99,000, and reduce the annual number of deaths from any cause by 44,000 to 92,000 in the United States (Bibbins-Domingo et al., 2010).
- It's also not a good idea to consume too little sodium because it is, in fact, a crucial electrolyte. According to a significant scientific study, eating too little salt can be even more harmful to your health than eating too much (Mente et al., 2016). Therefore, it's a good idea to cut back on your salt intake if you already consume too much of it, but you shouldn't go overboard. The best course of action while making such dietary adjustments is to consult a professional.

References

1. Bibbins-Domingo, K., Chertow, G. M., Coxson, P. G., Moran, A., Lightwood, J. M., Pletcher, M. J., & Goldman, L. (2010). Projected effect of dietary salt reductions on future cardiovascular disease. New England Journal of Medicine, 362(7), 590-599.
2. CDC. (2022, August 19). Sodium and Health. Centers for Disease Control and Prevention. https://www.cdc.gov/salt/index.htm
3. de Brito-Ashurst, I., Perry, L., Sanders, T. A., Thomas, J. E., Dobbie, H., Varagunam, M., & Yaqoob, M. M. (2013). The role of salt intake and salt sensitivity in the management of hypertension in South Asian people with chronic kidney disease: a randomised controlled trial. Heart, 99(17), 1256-1260.
4. He, J., Huang, J. F., Li, C., Chen, J., Lu, X., Chen, J. C., ... & Gu, D. F. (2021). Sodium sensitivity, Sodium resistance, and incidence of hypertension: a longitudinal follow-up study of dietary sodium intervention. Hypertension, 78(1), 155-164.
5. Hummel, S. L., Seymour, E. M., Brook, R. D., Kolias, T. J., Sheth, S. S., Rosenblum, H. R., ... & Weder, A. B. (2012). Low-sodium dietary approaches to stop hypertension diet reduces blood pressure, arterial

stiffness, and oxidative stress in hypertensive heart failure with preserved ejection fraction. Hypertension, 60(5), 1200-1206.

6. Mente, A., O'Donnell, M., Rangarajan, S., Dagenais, G., Lear, S., McQueen, M., et al. (2016). Associations of urinary sodium excretion with cardiovascular events in individuals with and without hypertension: a pooled analysis of data from four studies. The Lancet, 388(10043), 465-475.

7. Mu, L., Li, C., Liu, T., Xie, W., Li, G., Wang, M., ... & Wu, Y. (2020). A pilot study on efficacy and safety of a new salt substitute with very low sodium among hypertension patients on regular treatment. Medicine, 99(8).

8. Rahimdel, T., Morowatisharifabad, M. A., Salehi-Abargouei, A., Mirzaei, M., & Fallahzadeh, H. (2019). Evaluation of an education program based on the theory of planned behavior for salt intake in individuals at risk of hypertension. Health education research, 34(3), 268-278.

9. Yang, G. H., Zhou, X., Ji, W. J., Liu, J. X., Sun, J., Shi, R., ... & Li, Y. M. (2018). Effects of a low salt diet on isolated systolic hypertension: A community-based population study. Medicine, 97(14).

10. WHO, 2015, accessed: 17th May 2022, https://apps.who.int/iris/bitstream/handle/10665/155294/salt-factsheet-web.pdf

1.1.12 Beets

Participants in the experiment (Iranians with hypertension) described by Asgary et al. (2016) were given raw beet juice (RBJ) and cooked beets (CB) for 4 weeks. Blood pressure decreased in both groups, for raw beet juice by 6.67 mm Hg and for cooked beets by 5.41 mm Hg. The raw beetroot juice had greater antihypertensive effects. Since the effect did not exceed a reduction of more than 7 mm Hg, I will not describe the methodology in detail.

References

1. Asgary, S., Afshani, M. R., Sahebkar, A., Keshvari, M., Taheri, M., Jahanian, E., ... & Sarrafzadegan, N. (2016). Improvement of hypertension, endothelial function and systemic inflammation following short-term supplementation with red beet (Beta vulgaris L.) juice: a randomized crossover pilot study. Journal of human hypertension, 30(10), 627-632.

1.1.13 Seafood

Three papers describe how seafood impacted blood pressure (Izadi et al. 2020, Matsumoto et al. 2019, Minihane et al. 2016). Participants in the Minihane et al. (2016) trial consumed fish oil or a control oil containing 0.7 or 1.8 g of EPA+DHA (EPA - eicosapentaenoic acid, DHA - docosahexaenoic acid) per day for eight weeks. Among the different groups of subjects (normotensive, classic hypertensive, and isolated systolic hypertensive - ISH), the best effect was obtained in the ISH group where fish oil with 1.8 g EPA+DHA caused a mean decrease in blood pressure of 5.07 mm Hg, and 0.7 g EPA+DHA caused a mean decrease in blood pressure of 4.98 mm Hg. In the other groups there was even an increase in blood pressure relative to the beginning of the experiment.

Students were given 10 g (0.35 oz) of low-sodium seafood per day in the study by Izadi et al. (2020), which included fish filets of Atlantic salmon (Salmo salar) (50 percent) and tuna (50 percent). Blood pressure dropped by an average of 3.68 mm Hg after two months.

However, in the trial described in Matsumoto et al. (2019)'s paper, 12279 participants' blood pressure was measured together with their intake of omega-3 fatty acids. The studied data did not reveal any connections.

Since the data from the publications described above are not conclusive or the effect is small I will not go into their methodology.

References

1. Izadi, A., Khedmat, L., Tavakolizadeh, R., & Mojtahedi, S. Y. (2020). The intake assessment of diverse dietary patterns on childhood hypertension: alleviating the blood pressure and lipidemic factors with low-sodium seafood rich in omega-3 fatty acids. Lipids in health and disease, 19(1), 1-13.

2. Matsumoto, C., Yoruk, A., Wang, L., Gaziano, J. M., & Sesso, H. D. (2019). Fish and omega-3 fatty acid consumption and risk of hypertension. Journal of Hypertension, 37(6), 1223-1229.

3. Minihane, A. M., Armah, C. K., Miles, E. A., Madden, J. M., Clark, A. B., Caslake, M. J., ... & Calder, P. C. (2016). Consumption of fish oil providing amounts of eicosapentaenoic acid and docosahexaenoic acid that can be obtained from the diet reduces blood pressure in adults with systolic hypertension: a retrospective analysis. The Journal of Nutrition, 146(3), 516-523.

1.1.14 Spirulina sauce

In an 8-week investigation, Iranian volunteers regularly ate a vegetable salad with spirulina (Ghaem Far et al. 2021). They were split into four groups: those who had normal blood pressure, those who had high blood pressure (120 mm Hg $\leq$ systolic blood pressure (SBP) $\leq$ 130 mm Hg), those who had stage I hypertension (130 mm Hg $\leq$ SBP < 140 mm Hg), and those who had stage II hypertension (SBP $\geq$ 140 mm Hg). In the spirulina consumption group, it was discovered after the experiment that the number of individuals with stage II hypertension had been cut in half. Despite the paucity of data on the mean blood pressure readings before and after the experiment, it appears from the results that the intervention was very successful.

Spirulina - how was the intervention conducted?
The participants were instructed to top their daily vegetable salad with a 20 gram sachet of salad dressing (0.71 oz) that contained 2 grams of spirulina platensis powder (0.07 oz). This 10% dressing addition, according to the authors, was comparable to 2 g of pure spirulina (*Arthrospira platensis*) powder (0.07 oz).

2 grems per day → 8 weeks → 50%

* - the proportion of individuals who have stage II hypertension decreased by 50%

What you should know

- Spirulina may provide antioxidant, anti-inflammatory, and immune-boosting benefits.
- It is important to purchase spirulina from a reputable supplier since improperly cultivated algae can contain microcystins, which are particularly harmful to the liver (Dawson, 1998). These toxins could be present in up to 40% of products on

the market today in harmful amounts (Roy-Lachapelle et al., 2017).

- You should be careful with spirulina if you are taking blood thinners or have autoimmune diseases.
- Spirulina may cause mild side effects include headaches, sleeplessness, and nausea. However, this supplement is generally regarded as safe, and the majority of users report no negative effects (Ghaeni and Roomiani 2016).

References

1. Dawson, R. M. (1998). The toxicology of microcystins. Toxicon, 36(7), 953-962.
2. Ghaem Far, Z., Babajafari, S., Kojuri, J., Mohammadi, S., Nouri, M., Rostamizadeh, P., ... & Mazloomi, S. M. (2021). Antihypertensive and antihyperlipemic of spirulina (Arthrospira platensis) sauce on patients with hypertension: A randomized triple-blind placebo-controlled clinical trial. Phytotherapy Research, 35(11), 6181-6190.
3. Ghaeni, M., & Roomiani, L. (2016). Review for application and medicine effects of Spirulina, microalgae. Journal of Advanced Agricultural Technologies Vol, 3(2).
4. Roy-Lachapelle, A., Solliec, M., Bouchard, M. F., & Sauvé, S. (2017). Detection of cyanotoxins in algae dietary supplements. Toxins, 9(3), 76.

1.1.15 Summary of dietary interventions - what works

In conclusion, among the interventions examined, results for dairy products, the East Asian diet, gazpacho, the low-fat diet, miso soup, and seafood were either inconclusive or had a minimal effect. Of course, this does not imply that such a dietary adjustment has no impact on decreasing blood pressure. It only means that the reviewed publications did not find sufficient evidence to conclude that such an intervention is worthwhile. What works? According to the data from the analyzed publications, the highest blood pressure reduction was observed after implementation of the DASH diet, but not the classic one, but one modified by adaptation to the Japanese diet (reduced by 16.94-23 mm Hg), or combined with physical activity (reduced by 16.1-17.6 mm Hg) or significantly reduced amount of salt in the diet (reduced by 14.4-17 mm Hg). A comparable effect to following the DASH diet was produced by reducing salt by 50% (reduced by 12 mm Hg) or to 3g per day (0.11 oz)(reduced by 13.7 mm Hg) and eating oat bran (reduced by 15.3 mm Hg). Slightly less spectacular but no less promising results were obtained for the interventions of including beet juice (reduced by 6.67-8 mm Hg), olive oil (reduced by 7.91 mm Hg), blueberries (reduced by 7 mm Hg), and the addition of spirulina (50% fewer people with stage 2 hypertension) to the diet.

These results are presented graphically in Figure 3.

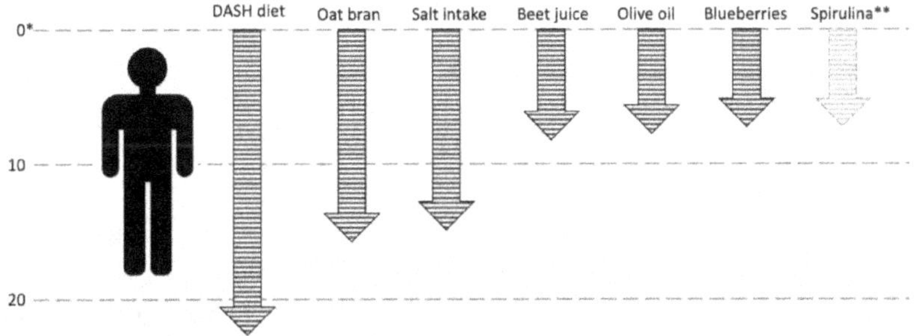

* - blood pressure reduction scale in units of mm Hg, which literally means the average of the highest systolic blood pressure reduction values reported in a given publication

** - the publication did not state by how much, on average, this intervention reduced blood pressure, but it is known to reduce the number of people with stage 2 hypertension

Figure 3. The most effective dietary interventions that affect blood pressure.

1.2 SUPPLEMENTATION

A review of 41 publications was the basis for this section. The effects of the following factors on blood pressure were examined over the ten years covered in this book:

- African traditional medicines (*Combretum micranthum* (kinkeliba) and *Hibiscus sabdariffa* (bissap))
- *Allium sativum* (garlic)
- American ginseng (*Panax quinquefolius*)
- Chios mastic
- Collagen
- Flaxseed
- Folic acid
- Fufang Danshen (*Salvia miltiorrhiza*)
- Ginseng
- Grape seed extract
- Green tea extract
- Indian kudzu
- L-arginine
- Lipoic acid (ALA)
- Magnesium
- *Melissa officinalis*
- Montmorency tart cherry
- Nigella sativa seed extract

- Omega-3
- Orthosiphon stamineus
- Peptides
- Selenium
- Quercetin (onion skin extract)
- Watermelon extract (L-citrulline/L-arginine)
- Vitamin B2
- Vitamin D
- Others (multicomponent supplementation)

The interventions that both seemed to lower blood pressure and those that were ineffective are summarized in Figure 4. After analyzing the different interventions, I include a summary showing the actual effect of supplementation at the end of this section.

Due to the absence of discernible effects, studies on L-arginine, Lipoic acid (ALA), *Nigella sativa* seed extract, and omega-3 fatty acids will not be presented.

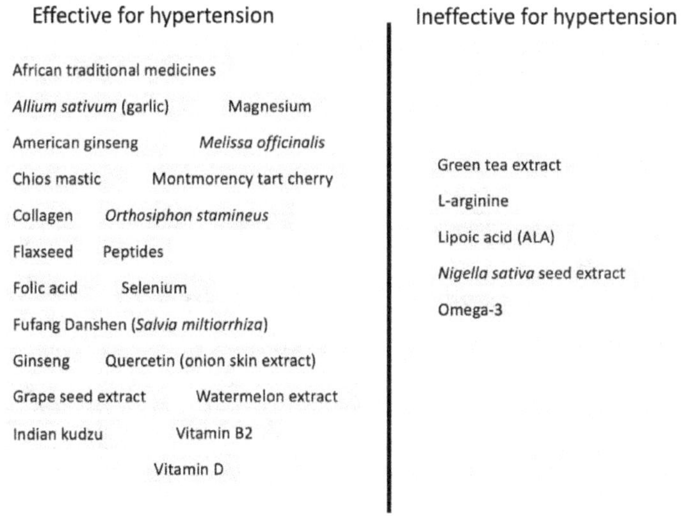

Figure 4. Comparison of different intervention strategies and their success or failure in reducing hypertension. The order of interventions is not determined by the outcome.

1.2.1 African herbs

According to Seck et al. (2018), 168 hypertensive Senegalese were divided into three groups and given capsules containing micronized powdered *Combretum micranthum* leaves (kinkeliba), *Hibiscus sabdariffa* (bissap calyx), and ramipril (a hypertension medication), respectively. The mean blood pressure dropped by 12.2 mm Hg in group 1, 11.2 mm Hg in group 2, and 16.7 mm Hg in group 3 after 4 weeks. The medication worked better, but supplements also significantly lowered blood pressure.

African herbs - how was the intervention conducted?
The individuals using capsules with *Combretum micranthum* leaves extract consumed 190 mg twice daily (380 mg total). Participants in the second group consumed 320 mg twice daily of *Hibiscus sabdariffa* calyx extract (640 mg total). The examination lasted four weeks.

A. 380 mg /day → 🧍 —————→ ↓12.2 mm Hg

4 weeks

B. 640 mg /day → 🧍 —————→ ↓11.2 mm Hg

What you should know
- *Combretum micranthum* (kinkeliba) and *Hibiscus sabdariffa* (bissap) are used to prepare beverages in West Africa.
- *Combretum micranthum*, also known as "kinkeliba," is largely used in Africa as a tea to treat hypertension. In certain African languages, "kinkeliba" is a synonym for "medicine" (Seck et al., 2018).
- Consuming kinkeliba and bissap may impact blood sugar levels; therefore, be cautious of interactions with medications having a similar effect (Welch et al., 2018).

- The absorption of chloroquine, a drug used in malaria, can be reduced in the presence of *Hibiscus sabdariffa*, so this combination should be avoided.
- Both plants' extracts and teas may interact with a variety of medications; if you intend to use them, remember to consult a professional first.

References

1. Seck, S. M., Doupa, D., Dia, D. G., Diop, E. A., Ardiet, D. L., Nogueira, R. C., ... & Diouf, B. (2018). Clinical efficacy of African traditional medicines in hypertension: A randomized controlled trial with Combretum micranthum and Hibiscus sabdariffa. Journal of Human Hypertension, 32(1), 75-81.
2. Seck, S. M., Doupa, D., Dia, D. G., Diop, E. A., Ardiet, D. L., Nogueira, R. C., ... & Diouf, B. (2018). Clinical efficacy of African traditional medicines in hypertension: a randomized controlled trial with Combretum micranthum and Hibiscus sabdariffa. Journal of human hypertension, 32(1), 75-81.
3. Welch, C., Zhen, J., Bassène, E., Raskin, I., Simon, J. E., & Wu, Q. (2018). Bioactive polyphenols in kinkéliba tea (Combretum micranthum) and their glucose-lowering activities. Journal of food and drug analysis, 26(2), 487-496.

1.2.2 *Allium sativum* (garlic)

Ashraf et al. (2013) administered garlic tablets to 150 individuals from Pakistan. A total of five different subject groups received daily doses of 300–1500 mg of garlic tablets. One group was a placebo and one group received the drug atenolol. According to the garlic dose, the experiment revealed blood pressure reductions in all subject groups ranging from 2.3 to 7.6 mm Hg. 9.2 mm Hg was the largest drop that was seen after taking the medication.

Allium sativum (garlic) - how was the intervention conducted?

Divided doses of 300 mg, 600 mg, 900 mg, 1200 mg, and 1500 mg were given to participants each day. However, there is no information on how these doses were divided. The experiment lasted 24 weeks. The blood pressure dropped by 2.3 mm Hg, 4.3 mm Hg, 6.1 mm Hg, 6.7 mm Hg, and 7.6 mm Hg in the groups consuming the garlic tablets, respectively.

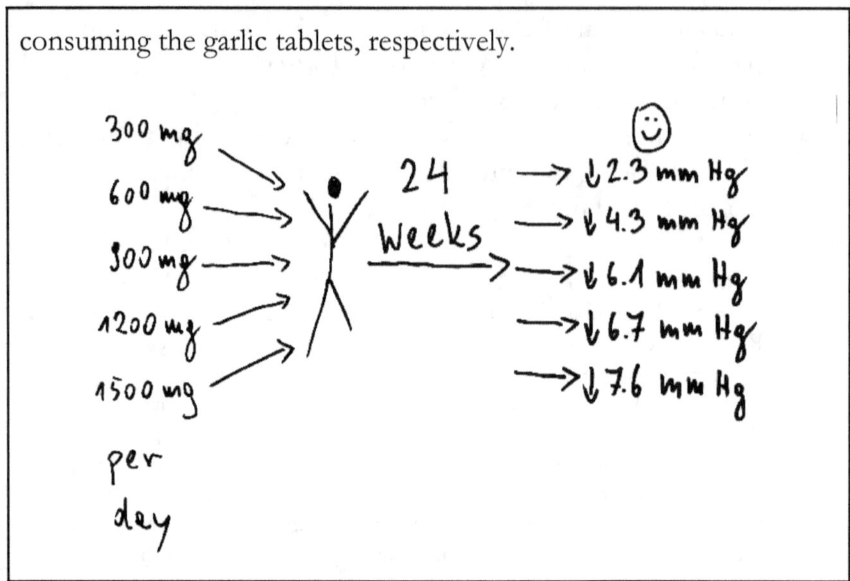

What you should know

- Allicin, which gives garlic its strong flavor and is thought to provide health benefits, is present in garlic. Therefore, some of the benefits of garlic may not be present in odorless formulations currently present on the market.
- Garlic can affect blood cholesterol levels, so be careful about using it with cholesterol-lowering medications.
- Garlic can have a beneficial effect on blood sugar levels, but you should be aware of the hazards when taking garlic along with drugs that lower blood sugar (Wang et al., 2017).
- Garlic has a variety of additional drug interactions, so it's a good idea to talk to your doctor before using garlic frequently, especially if you take any prescription medications.
- It's advised to avoid eating a lot of garlic, especially raw garlic, if you have severe acid reflux.

References

1. Ashraf, R., Khan, R. A., Ashraf, I., & Qureshi, A. A. (2013). Effects of Allium sativum (garlic) on systolic and diastolic blood pressure in patients with essential hypertension. Pakistan journal of pharmaceutical sciences, 26(5).
2. Wang, J., Zhang, X., Lan, H., & Wang, W. (2017). Effect of garlic supplement in the management of type 2 diabetes mellitus (T2DM): a

meta-analysis of randomized controlled trials. Food & nutrition research, 61(1), 1377571.

1.2.3 American ginseng (*Panax quinquefolius*)

According to Mucalo et al. (2013), study participants who supplemented with American ginseng experienced a drop in blood pressure of 17.4 mm Hg on average. The study included 64 individuals with simultaneous type 2 diabetes and hypertension.

> *American ginseng (Panax quinquefolius) - how was the intervention conducted?*
>
> The participants were instructed to take two 500 mg capsules of American ginseng extract (a total of three grams per day) three times each day, before each of their main meals. This extract had 10% of the total amount of ginsenosides that were extracted using ethanol. The experiment lasted for 12 weeks.
>
>

What you should know
- The fact that type 2 diabetics participated in this study may have had an impact on the results.
- As an alleged adaptogen, American ginseng has a variety of effects on the body, not necessarily in the ways we would expect (Szczuka et al., 2019)
- This article demonstrates the administration of a large dose. Regulators in several countries consider such a dose to be potentially excessive and do not permit the selling of such supplements.
- It is suspected that American ginseng may be unsafe to take during pregnancy.

- American ginseng and some medications used to treat depression have some known interactions.
- American ginseng may lower blood sugar levels, so drugs that impact blood sugar levels shouldn't be taken with it (Chen et al., 2019).
- It is best to see your doctor or other healthcare provider before deciding whether to take American ginseng supplements.

References

1. Chen, W., Balan, P., & Popovich, D. G. (2019). Review of ginseng anti-diabetic studies. Molecules, 24(24), 4501.
2. Mucalo, I., Jovanovski, E., Rahelić, D., Božikov, V., Romić, Ž., & Vuksan, V. (2013). Effect of American ginseng (Panax quinquefolius L.) on arterial stiffness in subjects with type-2 diabetes and concomitant hypertension. Journal of ethnopharmacology, 150(1), 148-153.
3. Szczuka, D., Nowak, A., Zakłos-Szyda, M., Kochan, E., Szymańska, G., Motyl, I., & Blasiak, J. (2019). American ginseng (Panax quinquefolium L.) as a source of bioactive phytochemicals with pro-health properties. Nutrients, 11(5), 1041.

1.2.4 Chios mastic

Chios mastic, a resin of *Pistacia lentiscus* var. *chia*, was supplemented in an experiment described by Kontogiannis et al. (2019). In Greek participants who were hypertensive, the intervention reduced blood pressure by an average of 9 mm Hg 3 hours after taking the supplement, but it had no effect on those who were normotensive (individuals who do not have hypertension).

Chios mastic - how was the intervention conducted?

Participants underwent two visits, consuming four tablets each containing 700 mg of chios mastic for a total of 2800 mg. Three hours after taking the supplement, the effects mentioned above were achieved.

2800 mg total → 3 hours → 9 mm Hg

What you should know

- An allergy to pistachios can also mean an allergy to chios mastic.
- Mastic gum has been demonstrated to improve digestion and even lessen the amount of *Helicobacter pylori* in the stomach (Dabos et al., 2010).
- Mastic gum may lower cholesterol and blood glucose levels (Kartalis et al., 2016). For this reason, you should be careful about taking medications that have a similar effect at the same time.
- Mastic gum shouldn't be consumed if you are pregnant or breastfeeding.

References

1. Dabos, K. J., Sfika, E., Vlatta, L. J., & Giannikopoulos, G. (2010). The effect of mastic gum on Helicobacter pylori: a randomized pilot study. Phytomedicine, 17(3-4), 296-299.
2. Kartalis, A., Didagelos, M., Georgiadis, I., Benetos, G., Smyrnioudis, N., Marmaras, H., ... & Andrikopoulos, G. (2016). Effects of Chios mastic gum on cholesterol and glucose levels of healthy volunteers: A prospective, randomized, placebo-controlled, pilot study (CHIOS-MASTIHA). European journal of preventive cardiology, 23(7), 722-729.
3. Kontogiannis, C., Georgiopoulos, G., Loukas, K., Papanagnou, E. D., Pachi, V. K., Bakogianni, I., ... & Stamatelopoulos, K. (2019). Chios mastic improves blood pressure haemodynamics in patients with arterial hypertension: Implications for regulation of proteostatic pathways. European Journal of Preventive Cardiology, 26(3), 328-331.

1.2.5 Collagen

In a study published by Kouguchi et al. (2013), 58 Japanese subjects were examined for 12 weeks to see how chicken collagen hydrolysate affected their blood pressure. After this time, there was an average drop in blood pressure of 9.3 mm Hg.

Collagen - how was the intervention conducted?

A lactic acid beverage (120 ml) containing 2.9 grams of chicken collagen hydrolysate (0.01 oz) was consumed by participants every day.. It appears that this kind of beverage was selected to ensure that neither the control group nor the test group would know whether or not the beverage included collagen.

What you should know

- There are as many as 28 different kinds of collagen. The function of collagen differs depending on where it comes from. Marine collagen may help skin and cartilage health, while chicken collagen may help reduce inflammation and be connected to joint, cartilage, and ligament health. Bovine collagen is known to be helpful for skin elasticity and hydration.
- You should stay away from chicken collagen if you have an egg or chicken allergy.
- Chicken collagen contains chondroitin and glucosamine, commonly used in treating the joint diseases (Vasiliadis and Tsikopoulos, 2017).
- Chicken soup, bone broth, and chicken feet are rich in chicken collagen.

References

1. Kouguchi, T., Ohmori, T., Shimizu, M., Takahata, Y., Maeyama, Y., Suzuki, T., ... & Tanabe, S. (2013). Effects of a chicken collagen hydrolysate on the circulation system in subjects with mild hypertension or high-normal blood pressure. Bioscience, biotechnology, and biochemistry, 77(4), 691-696.

2.   Vasiliadis, H. S., & Tsikopoulos, K. (2017). Glucosamine and chondroitin for the treatment of osteoarthritis. World journal of orthopedics, 8(1), 1.

1.2.6 Flaxseed

In the experiment detailed by Caligiuri et al. (2014), individuals from Canada who were 75% hypertensive and had peripheral artery disease took milled flaxseed for 6 months, which led to an average 10 mm Hg reduction in blood pressure.

Flaxseed - how was the intervention conducted?
For 6 months, participants consumed food products containing 30 g of milled flaxseed daily (1.06 oz).

What you should know
- Participants with peripheral arterial disease enrolled in this experiment, which may have had an impact on the results.
- A tablespoon of flaxseed oil contains 7 grams of omega-3 fats (0.25 oz), which are then converted by the body into about 700 milligrams (mg) of EPA and DHA (conversion occurs with an efficiency of 10-15%). This is a pretty good source of omega-3 fatty acids (Harvard Medical School website, 2019).
- Flaxseed is the richest known source of lignans (9–30 mg per gram), which prevent and alleviate lifestyle-related diseases (Imran et al., 2015).
- However, due to the presence of cyanogenic glycosides in this plant, which emit harmful hydrogen cyanide in the presence of water, ingesting raw or unripe flaxseed may be dangerous. According to a report by the European Food Safety Authority (EFSA), youngsters can already be at risk with just one-third of a teaspoon of tea, compared to three

tablespoons for adults (EFSA, 2019). Be cautious; it's better to seek a specialist's advice before taking such supplements.

References

1. Caligiuri, S. P., Aukema, H. M., Ravandi, A., Guzman, R., Dibrov, E., & Pierce, G. N. (2014). Flaxseed consumption reduces blood pressure in patients with hypertension by altering circulating oxylipins via an α-linolenic acid–induced inhibition of soluble epoxide hydrolase. Hypertension, 64(1), 53-59.
2. EFSA Panel on Contaminants in the Food Chain (CONTAM), Schrenk, D., Bignami, M., Bodin, L., Chipman, J. K., del Mazo, J., ... & Schwerdtle, T. (2019). Evaluation of the health risks related to the presence of cyanogenic glycosides in foods other than raw apricot kernels. EFSA Journal, 17(4), e05662.
3. Harvard Medical School, Why not flaxseed oil? - Harvard Health. (2006, October 1). Harvard Health. https://www.health.harvard.edu/heart-health/why-not-flaxseed-oil
4. Imran, M., Ahmad, N., Anjum, F. M., Khan, M. K., Mushtaq, Z., Nadeem, M., & Hussain, S. (2015). Potential protective properties of flax lignan secoisolariciresinol diglucoside. Nutrition journal, 14(1), 1-7.

1.2.7 Folic acid

Genotype-specific folic acid supplementation was tested on Chinese participants (Zhang et al. 2022). A mean blood pressure reduction of 2.6 mm Hg was achieved. Since this was not a meaningful effect, I will not go into a description of the methodology.

References

1. Zhang, S., Wang, T., Wang, H., Tang, J., Hou, A., Yan, X., ... & He, H. (2022). Effects of individualized administration of folic acid on prothrombotic state and vascular endothelial function with H-type hypertension: A double-blinded, randomized clinical cohort study. Medicine, 101(3).

1.2.8 Fufang Danshen

Taiwanese hypertension patients were supplemented with Fufang Danshen capsules, which comprised Danshen, *Rhodiola rosea*, *Chrysanthemum*, and *Pueraria* extract, according to a study by Yang et al. (2012). The blood pressure dropped by 13.8 mm Hg in comparison to the control group after 12 weeks.

> ### *Fufang Danshen - how was the intervention conducted?*
> Participants took a Fufang Danshen capsule (formula mixture) 500 mg twice-daily (1000 mg in total), which contained 225 mg purified Danshen extract, mixed with 20 mg *Rhodiola rosea* extract, 100 mg *Chrysanthemum* extract, and 100 mg *Pueraria* extract.
>
> 1000 mg per day → 12 weeks → 13.8 mm Hg

What you should know

- Herbs are used in the above-mentioned intervention, so use caution due to their interactions with medicines and diseases. Before undergoing such interventions, consulting a specialist is recommended.
- Danshen appears to thin the blood, therefore use caution when undergoing surgery or using drugs that have comparable effects.
- *Rhodiola rosea* is a so-called adaptogen, it can influence the human body in many ways, not always the way we would like (Hung et al., 2011).
- Chrysanthemum extract may increase sensitivity to insulin (Chen et al., 2019).
- A phytochemical found in chrysanthemum called alantolactone greatly increases the skin's sensitivity to sunlight (Paulsen and Andersen, 2020).

References

1. Chen, M., Wang, K., Zhang, Y., Zhang, M., Ma, Y., Sun, H., ... & Sun, H. (2019). New insights into the biological activities of Chrysanthemum morifolium: Natural flavonoids alleviate diabetes by targeting α-glucosidase and the PTP-1B signaling pathway. European Journal of Medicinal Chemistry, 178, 108-115.
2. Hung, S. K., Perry, R., & Ernst, E. (2011). The effectiveness and efficacy of Rhodiola rosea L.: a systematic review of randomized clinical trials. Phytomedicine, 18(4), 235-244.

3. Paulsen, E., & Andersen, K. E. (2020). Contact sensitization to florists' chrysanthemums and marguerite daisies in Denmark: A 21-year experience. Contact Dermatitis, 82(1), 18-23.
4. Yang, T. Y., Wei, J. C. C., Lee, M. Y., Chen, C. B., & Ueng, K. C. (2012). A Randomized, Double-blind, Placebo-controlled Study to Evaluate the Efficacy and Tolerability of Fufang Danshen (Salvia miltiorrhiza) as Add-on Antihypertensive Therapy in Taiwanese Patients with Uncontrolled Hypertension. Phytotherapy Research, 26(2), 291-298.

1.2.9 Ginseng

Jovanovski et al. (2020) evaluated the combination of two ginseng species—American ginseng and Korean Red ginseng—over a 12-week period on individuals from Canada and Croatia who had type 2 diabetes and hypertension. At the end of the experiment, there was a statistically significant reduction in blood pressure (specifically end-systolic pressure) of 6.6 mm Hg. And since end-systolic pressure = 0.9 × systolic blood pressure, the reduction was probably about 7.3 mm Hg.

Ginseng - how was the intervention conducted?

Participants in this experiment took 1.5 grams per day of American ginseng (the preparation contained 10% ginsensoides) and 0.75 grams per day of Korean Red ginseng (the preparation contained 30% ginsensoides). The participants' task was to supplement these doses and divide them into 3 servings per day. In addition, Korean Red ginseng was fortified with ginsenoside Rg3. In total, participants took 75 mg of ginsenoside Rg3 and 375 mg of total ginsenosides each day.

What you should know

- Both Korean red ginseng (*Panax ginseng*) and American ginseng (*Panax quinquefolius*) are adaptogens that have a variety of physiological effects and may interact with a wide range of medications.

- American ginseng can lower blood sugar levels so you need to be careful about interacting with medications with similar effects.

- Ginseng shouldn't be used while pregnant because there are concerns that it could cause birth abnormalities (Kim et al., 2013).

- Ginseng has many different effects, therefore taking supplements should be reviewed with a medical expert beforehand.

References

1. Jovanovski, E., Komishon, A., Au-Yeung, F., Zurbau, A., Jenkins, A. L., Sung, M. K., ... & Vuksan, V. (2020). Vascular effects of combined enriched Korean Red ginseng (Panax Ginseng) and American ginseng (Panax Quinquefolius) administration in individuals with hypertension and type 2 diabetes: A randomized controlled trial. Complementary Therapies in Medicine, 49, 102338.

2. Kim, P., Park, J. H., Kwon, K. J., Kim, K. C., Kim, H. J., Lee, J. M., ... & Shin, C. Y. (2013). Effects of Korean red ginseng extracts on neural tube defects and impairment of social interaction induced by prenatal exposure to valproic acid. Food and chemical toxicology, 51, 288-296.

1.2.10 Grape seed extract

There are two articles that discuss the impact of grape seed extract on blood pressure in the ten-year period under consideration. In one study, participants received 300 mg of the extract in the form of capsules (Ras et al. 2013), and in the other, the same dosage was administered as juice (Park et al. 2016). It's interesting to note that while the blood pressure was only dropped by an average of 3 mm Hg in the first publication, it was already reduced by 9 mm Hg in the second. The methodology from the paper with the stronger effect is presented below, along with a comparison to the methodology from the publication with the smaller effect.

Grape seed extract - how was the intervention conducted?

In two daily dosages of 150 mg each, Park et al. (2016) provided participants with 300 mg of grape seed extract in the form of an apple, red grape, pomegranate, and raspberry fruit juice blend with the extract added. Over the period of six weeks, the individuals were instructed to drink the juice once in the morning and once in the evening, preferably with meals. Additionally, participants were instructed to continue with their current life style, level of activity, and nutrition. Participants in the second publication, where the effect was less beneficial, took 300 mg of grape seed extract in a capsule after breakfast. Additionally, they were instructed to limit their consumption of red fruit and tea to two servings each per day and to keep away from items high in polyphenols such as dark chocolate, red wine, and grape juice.

What you should know

- Grape seed extract lower the levels of cholesterol and should not be taken with similarly acting medications.
- Red grape varieties are likely to contain the most antioxidants, compared to others.
- Grape seed proanthocyanidin extracts are among the most powerful antioxidants, with antioxidant activity 50 times greater than that of vitamin E and 20 times greater than that of vitamin C (Gao et al., 2018).

References

1. Gao, Z., Liu, G., Hu, Z., Shi, W., Chen, B., Zou, P., & Li, X. (2018). Grape seed proanthocyanidins protect against streptozotocin-induced diabetic nephropathy by attenuating endoplasmic reticulum stress-induced apoptosis. Molecular Medicine Reports, 18(2), 1447-1454.

2. Park, E., Edirisinghe, I., Choy, Y. Y., Waterhouse, A., & Burton-Freeman, B. (2016). Effects of grape seed extract beverage on blood pressure and metabolic indices in individuals with pre-hypertension: a randomised, double-blinded, two-arm, parallel, placebo-controlled trial. British Journal of Nutrition, 115(2), 226-238.

3. Ras, R. T., Zock, P. L., Zebregs, Y. E., Johnston, N. R., Webb, D. J., & Draijer, R. (2013). Effect of polyphenol-rich grape seed extract on ambulatory blood pressure in subjects with pre-and stage I hypertension. British Journal of Nutrition, 110(12), 2234-2241.

1.2.11 Green tea

Women who participated in a 6-week experiment were split into 4 groups, and the effects of green tea drinking and exercise on blood pressure were noticed in each group (Taati et al. 2021). While resistance training can lower blood pressure by as much as 15 mm Hg, drinking green tea lowers it by around 5 mm Hg. The group that drank green tea and did resistance exercise saw an average drop in blood pressure of 14.09 mm Hg from the beginning of the trial. Since the reduced effect in the "green tea group" is not greater than 7 mm Hg, I will not go into depth regarding the methodology.

References

1. Taati, B., Arazi, H., & Kheirkhah, J. (2021). Interaction effect of green tea consumption and resistance training on office and ambulatory cardiovascular parameters in women with high-normal/stage 1 hypertension. The Journal of Clinical Hypertension, 23(5), 978-986.

1.2.12 Indian kudzu (*Pueraria tuberosa*)

Indian participants consumed 3 grams (0.11 oz) of *Pueraria tuberosa* tubers each day for 12 weeks (Verma et al. 2012). It had a spectacular effect, lowering individuals' stage 1 (primary) hypertension blood pressure by an average of 25 mm Hg.

Indian kudzu - how was the intervention conducted?

As a demonstration, the tubers were manually prepared. They were divided into little pieces and dried in the shade at room

---

temperature. They were then put in capsules after being mechanically ground into powder. There was 0.75 grams of powder in each pill. Participants took two pills twice daily. The publication omits any additional information.

3 grams per day → 🧍 — 12 weeks → 25 mm Hg 😊😊😊 ⬇

What you should know

- Kudzu could be used to treat alcoholism and alleviate the effects of a hangover (Penetar et al., 2015). The findings in this regard, however, are not conclusive.
- Kudzu should not be combined with medications that have comparable side effects since it can drop blood sugar levels and slow blood coagulation.
- Kudzu may lessen the effectiveness of birth control pills when taken together.

References

1. Penetar, D. M., Toto, L. H., Lee, D. Y. W., & Lukas, S. E. (2015). A single dose of kudzu extract reduces alcohol consumption in a binge drinking paradigm. Drug and alcohol dependence, 153, 194-200.
2. Verma, S. K., Jain, V., & Singh, D. P. (2012). Effect of Pueraria tuberosa DC.(Indian Kudzu) on blood pressure, fibrinolysis and oxidative stress in patients with stage 1 hypertension. Pakistan journal of biological sciences: PJBS, 15(15), 742-747.

1.2.13 Magnesium

Serbian participants received magnesium supplements for one month, according to Banjanin and Belojevic (2018). Following this period, the blood pressure of patients with essential hypertension was observed to drop by an average of 8.97 mm Hg.

> ***Magnesium - how was the intervention conducted?***
> For one month, participants took a daily dosage of 300 mg of magnesium oxide.
>
> 300 mg per day → 🧍 —month→ 8.97 mm Hg 🙂 ⇓

What you should know

- Excessive alcohol consumption can lead to magnesium deficiency (Abbott et al., 1994). Magnesium deficiency is also associated with the development of insulin resistance (Chaudhary et al., 2010)
- By boosting medicine absorption, for instance, magnesium supplementation may have an impact on how various substances are absorbed. Talk to a professional about your intention of taking magnesium supplements.
- Magnesium oxide - this form of magnesium is considered to be one of the least absorbable by the body, yet in the publication discussed above it was found to be effective in lowering blood pressure. Magnesium citrate, magnesium acetyl taurate, magnesium malate, and magnesium glycinate all have high absorption rates (Blancquaert et al., 2019).
- Magnesium oxide may reduce migraines in children and adults (Karimi et al., 2021; Wang et al., 2003).

References

1. Abbott, L., Nadler, J., & Rude, R. K. (1994). Magnesium deficiency in alcoholism: possible contribution to osteoporosis and cardiovascular disease in alcoholics. Alcoholism: Clinical and Experimental Research, 18(5), 1076-1082.
2. Banjanin, N., & Belojevic, G. (2018). Changes of blood pressure and hemodynamic parameters after oral magnesium supplementation in patients with essential hypertension—an intervention study. Nutrients, 10(5), 581.
3. Blancquaert, L., Vervaet, C., & Derave, W. (2019). Predicting and testing bioavailability of magnesium supplements. Nutrients, 11(7), 1663.

4. Chaudhary, D. P., Sharma, R., & Bansal, D. D. (2010). Implications of magnesium deficiency in type 2 diabetes: a review. Biological trace element research, 134(2), 119-129.
5. Karimi, N., Razian, A., & Heidari, M. (2021). The efficacy of magnesium oxide and sodium valproate in prevention of migraine headache: a randomized, controlled, double-blind, crossover study. Acta Neurologica Belgica, 121(1), 167-173.
6. Wang, F., Van Den Eeden, S. K., Ackerson, L. M., Salk, S. E., Reince, R. H., & Elin, R. J. (2003). Oral magnesium oxide prophylaxis of frequent migrainous headache in children: a randomized, double-blind, placebo-controlled trial. Headache: The Journal of Head and Face Pain, 43(6), 601-610.

1.2.14 *Melissa officinalis*

Iranians with stage 1 essential hypertension completed a 4-week trial of *Melissa officinalis* supplementation (Shekarriz et al. 2021). Throughout the experiment, they kept taking their hypertension medication. At the end of the experiment, they found that their blood pressure was reduced by as much as 21.45 mm Hg on average.

Melissa officinalis - how was the intervention conducted?

Study participants consumed capsules containing 400 mg of Melissa officinalis extract three times a day (1200 mg total) for 4 weeks, one after each meal. According to the authors, this 70% hydroalcoholic extract contained 8 mg of rosmarinic acid, corn starch, lactose monohydrate (milk sugar), magnesium acetate, and alpha-tocopherol.

What you should know

- One of the described effects of *Melissa officinalis* supplementation was an increase in appetite (Świąder et al., 2019).

- If you have a thyroid condition, avoid using *Melissa officinalis* supplements without first consulting your doctor. They may have an adverse effect on the thyroid gland.
- Supplementing with *Melissa officinalis* may make you sleepy and make you breathe more slowly. Therefore, it is not recommended when taking sedative medications.

References

1. Shekarriz, Z., Shorofi, S. A., Nabati, M., Shabankhani, B., & Yousefi, S. S. (2021). Effect of Melissa officinalis on systolic and diastolic blood pressures in essential hypertension: A double-blind crossover clinical trial. Phytotherapy Research, 35(12), 6883-6892.
2. Świąder, K., Startek, K., & Wijaya, C. H. (2019). The therapeutic properties of Lemon balm (Melissa officinalis L.): Reviewing novel findings and medical indications. J. Appl. Bot. Food Qual, 92, 327-335.

1.2.15 Montmorency tart cherry (*Prunus cerasus*)

Keane et al. (2016) describe a single Montmorency tart cherry concentrate supplementation, following which participants' blood pressure was recorded hourly. Participating in the study were 15 early-onset hypertensive men from the United Kingdom. It was discovered that this kind of intervention lowers blood pressure, with the biggest drop occurring two hours after the intervention at a reduction of roughly 7 mm Hg.

Montmorency tart cherry - how was the intervention conducted?

One dose of 60 mL of Montmorency tart cherry concentrate was given to each participant, who then drank it after diluting it with 100 mL of water. This is comparable to roughly 180 cherries, according to the concentrate's producer.

$$60 \text{ mL} \longrightarrow \overset{2}{\underset{}{\text{hours}}} \longrightarrow 7 \text{ mm Hg} \downarrow$$

$$= 180 \text{ cherries}$$

What you should know

- Cherry fruit contains melatonin and appears to have the potential to regulate sleep patterns (Zhao et al., 2013).
- Natural anti-inflammatory substances are present in cherry fruits (Kuehl, 2012). Researchers discovered a link between drinking tart cherry juice and reduced blood levels of high sensitivity C-reactive protein (hsCRP), a protein that can signify inflammation in the body (Hanna et al. 2008).
- Cherry eating may lessen the muscular damage caused by exercise and enhance athletic performance (Ferretti et al., 2010).

References

1. Ferretti, G., Bacchetti, T., Belleggia, A., & Neri, D. (2010). Cherry antioxidants: from farm to table. Molecules, 15(10), 6993-7005.
2. Hanna, F. S., Bell, R. J., Cicuttini, F. M., Davison, S. L., Wluka, A. E., & Davis, S. R. (2008). High sensitivity C-reactive protein is associated with lower tibial cartilage volume but not lower patella cartilage volume in healthy women at mid-life. Arthritis research & therapy, 10(1), 1-7.
3. Keane, K. M., George, T. W., Constantinou, C. L., Brown, M. A., Clifford, T., & Howatson, G. (2016). Effects of Montmorency tart cherry (Prunus Cerasus L.) consumption on vascular function in men with early hypertension. The American journal of clinical nutrition, 103(6), 1531-1539.
4. Kuehl, K. S. (2012). Cherry juice targets antioxidant potential and pain relief. Acute Topics in Sport Nutrition, 59, 86-93.
5. Zhao, Y., Tan, D. X., Lei, Q., Chen, H., Wang, L., Li, Q. T., ... & Kong, J. (2013). Melatonin and its potential biological functions in the fruits of sweet cherry. Journal of Pineal Research, 55(1), 79-88.

1.2.16 *Orthosiphon stamineus*

The effects of Orthosiphon stamineus on blood pressure were examined in Italian participants with grade 1 essential hypertension as described by Trimarco et al. (2012). An average drop in blood pressure of more than 15 mm Hg was seen after 4 weeks.

> ### *Orthosiphon stamineus - how was the intervention conducted?*
> The combination of policosanol, red yeast rice extract, berberine, folic acid and coenzyme Q(10) with or without *Orthosiphon stamineus* in a ratio of 2 : 1 was used. Unfortunately, there is not enough information available on the dosages, application techniques, and forms of the supplement components.

What you should know

- *Orthosiphon stamineus* leaves are known as "Java tea" and are used for making herbal tea in Southeast Asia and European countries (Ashraf et al., 2018).
- The amount of water expelled in urine could be increased by java tea (diuretic effect). Be careful with concomitant use with medications with similar effects.
- Java tea can reduce cholesterol, therefore also be cautious of interactions with drugs that have equivalent effects. (Maheswari et al., 2015).

References

1. Ashraf, K., Sultan, S., & Adam, A. (2018). Orthosiphon stamineus Benth. is an outstanding food medicine: Review of phytochemical and pharmacological activities. Journal of pharmacy & bioallied sciences, 10(3), 109.
2. Maheswari, C., Venkatnarayanan, R., Babu, P., & Kandasamy, C. S. (2015). Green tea (cardiac tea) vs java tea (kidney tea): A review. Research Journal of Pharmacy and Technology, 8(1), 94-100.
3. Trimarco, V., Cimmino, C. S., Santoro, M., Pagnano, G., Manzi, M. V., Piglia, A., ... & Izzo, R. (2012). Nutraceuticals for blood pressure control in patients with high-normal or grade 1 hypertension. High Blood Pressure & Cardiovascular Prevention, 19(3), 117-122.

1.2.17 Peptides

The use of peptides* (Isoleucine-Proline-Proline/Valine-Proline-Proline) as supplements was evaluated in Italian participants with normal blood pressure or first-degree hypertension (Cicero et al. 2012). The experiment's results were inconclusive after 6 weeks; no effect was seen for ambulatory blood pressure, but office blood pressure was somewhat reduced, on average by 3.42 mm Hg. In relation to the findings, I will not go into detail about the experiment's methods.

* - short strands of amino acids connected by peptide bonds are called peptidides.

References

1. Cicero, A. F. G., Rosticci, M., Ferroni, A., Bacchelli, S., Veronesi, M., Strocchi, E., & Borghi, C. (2012). Predictors of the short-term effect of Isoleucine–Proline–Proline/Valine–Proline–Proline Lactotripeptides from casein on office and ambulatory blood pressure in subjects with pharmacologically untreated high-normal blood pressure or first-degree hypertension. Clinical and experimental hypertension, 34(8), 601-605.

1.2.18 Selenium

In a study published by Wu et al. (2018), more than 9,000 Chinese participants underwent testing to determine whether blood selenium levels were connected to blood pressure. It was interesting to discover that the risk of hypertension increased by 19% at the highest selenium levels. This interaction was only observed in women. The average level of high blood selenium concentrations, according to the authors of this study, is 155.84 g/l (standard deviation: ± 13.73 g/l).

References

1. Wu, G., Li, Z., Ju, W., Yang, X., Fu, X., & Gao, X. (2018). Cross-sectional study: relationship between serum selenium and hypertension in the Shandong Province of China. Biological trace element research, 185(2), 295-301.

1.2.19 Quercetin

Three papers have discussed quercetin supplementation; two of the studies were conducted in Germany and one in Ukraine. When an experiment was conducted on overweight-to-obese hypertension individuals, Brüll et al. (2017) reported no effects from supplementation; however, Ukrainian researchers reported a drop of up to 19.5 mm Hg on average after 12 months of intense supplementation (Kondratiuk and Synytsia 2018). In contrast, supplementation documented by Brüll et al. (2015) for 6 weeks led to a minor but statistically significant drop in blood pressure by an average of 3.6 mm Hg. This study was published two years prior to the first publication listed above (same authors).

Quercetin - how was the intervention conducted?

Patients with gout and essential hypertension were treated with quercetin at doses of 1000 mg twice daily for 30 minutes before meals for the first six months, followed by 500 mg twice daily for an additional six months, in the study by Kondratiuk and Synytsia (2018). For overweight-to-obese patients with pre-hypertension and stage I hypertension, Brüll et al. (2015) administered a much lower dose. Only in the hypertensive patients did the minor impact mentioned above appear after 6 weeks of taking 162 mg daily. An even smaller dose of 54 mg was applied in an experiment where no noticeable effects were observed (Brüll et al. 2017).

What you should know

- Quercetin is a plant pigment that can be found in red wine, onions, green tea, apples, berries, Ginkgo biloba, St. John's wort, and others.
- Quercetin is generally considered safe, although supplementing with quercetin might occasionally cause headaches or tingling in the arms and legs (Wieslander et al., 2012).

- There are several pharmacological interactions with quercetin, so it is strongly advised that you consult your doctor before supplementing.

References

1. Brüll, V., Burak, C., Stoffel-Wagner, B., Wolffram, S., Nickenig, G., Müller, C., ... & Egert, S. (2017). Acute intake of quercetin from onion skin extract does not influence postprandial blood pressure and endothelial function in overweight-to-obese adults with hypertension: a randomized, double-blind, placebo-controlled, crossover trial. European journal of nutrition, 56(3), 1347-1357.
2. Brüll, V., Burak, C., Stoffel-Wagner, B., Wolffram, S., Nickenig, G., Müller, C., ... & Egert, S. (2015). Effects of a quercetin-rich onion skin extract on 24 h ambulatory blood pressure and endothelial function in overweight-to-obese patients with (pre-) hypertension: a randomised double-blinded placebo-controlled cross-over trial. British Journal of Nutrition, 114(8), 1263-1277.
3. Kondratiuk, V. E., & Synytsia, Y. P. (2018). Effect of quercetin on the echocardiographic parameters of left ventricular diastolic function in patients with gout and essential hypertension. Wiadomosci lekarskie (Warsaw, Poland : 1960), 71(8), 1554–1559.
4. Wieslander, G., Fabjan, N., Vogrincic, M., Kreft, I., Vombergar, B., & Norbäck, D. (2012). Effects of common and Tartary buckwheat consumption on mucosal symptoms, headache and tiredness: A double-blind crossover intervention study. Journal of Food, Agriculture & Environment (JFAE), 10(2), 107-110.

1.2.20 Vitamin B2 (riboflavin)

In an experiment described by Wilson et al. (2012), participants who were homozygous for the MTHFR gene 677C/T polymorphism (TT genotype) were given vitamin B2 supplements. The experiment was carried out because prior research demonstrated that these individuals are more prone to have hypertension and have much higher homocysteine levels, which have a detrimental effect on the circulatory system. The intervention reduced blood pressure by 9.2 mm Hg on average.

Vitamin B2 - how was the intervention conducted?
For 16 weeks, patients with cardiovascular disease in Britain received 1.6 mg of vitamin B2 daily.

What you should know

- The aforementioned experiment was carried out on people who shared a particular genotype, which accounts for around 20% of the population. It's possible that people with different genotypes won't see this kind of considerable blood pressure reduction.
- Urine may appear more yellow than usual when riboflavin is taken, especially in high dosages.
- Tetracycline antibiotics may become less effective when riboflavin is administered.
- Vitamin B2 deficiency is very uncommon.
- Riboflavin supplementation could possibly reduce the risk of diabetes complications (Thakur et al., 2017).

References

1. Thakur, K., Tomar, S. K., Singh, A. K., Mandal, S., & Arora, S. (2017). Riboflavin and health: a review of recent human research. Critical reviews in food science and nutrition, 57(17), 3650-3660.
2. Wilson, C. P., Ward, M., McNulty, H., Strain, J. J., Trouton, T. G., Horigan, G., ... & Scott, J. M. (2012). Riboflavin offers a targeted strategy for managing hypertension in patients with the MTHFR 677TT genotype: a 4-y follow-up. The American journal of clinical nutrition, 95(3), 766-772.

1.2.21 Vitamin D

As many as 11 publications address the association between vitamin D and blood pressure (Alpsoy et al. 2016, Arora et al. 2015, Chen et al. 2014, de Paula et al. 2020, Larsen et al. 2012, Panahi et al. 2021, Sheikh et al. 2020, Wang et al. 2013, Witham et al. 2013, Witham et al. 2014a, Witham et al. 2014b). However, the results are not conclusive. In 4 publications no effect was found, in another two the effect depended on how the measurements were conducted. A reduction in blood pressure of more than 7 mm Hg was observed in only two publications.

Two publications out of these eleven analyzed the association between blood levels of vitamin D metabolites and the occurrence of hypertension, but these studies were non-interventional (Alpsoy et al. 2016, Wang et al. 2013). Both demonstrated the existence of such an association. The study, which lasted more than 15 years, is described by Wang et al. (2013), and involved observing just over 1,200 American men, more than 600 of whom developed hypertension during the experiment. After examining blood levels of vitamin D metabolites, it was found that the group with 30-40 ng/mL (75-100 nmol/L) of vitamin D in their blood had the lowest risk. A somewhat similar study was reported by Alpsoy et al. (2016), where it was found that Turkish individuals suffering from hypertension had an average of 26.4 ng/mL of vitamin D in their blood, while healthy individuals had 36 ng/mL.

Vitamin D - how was the intervention conducted?

Given the high level of interest in vitamin D supplementation, I chose to outline all the methodologies.

In a study by de Paula et al. (2020), vitamin D's effect on blood pressure was measured 8 weeks after administration in Brazilian patients with type 2 diabetes, hypertension, and hypovitaminosis D (25(OH) D serum concentration below 20 ng/mL or 50 nmol/L). The best effect was obtained with a reduction in blood pressure of up to 7.5 mm Hg.

Chinese patients with grades I-II essential hypertension were given 2000 IU of vitamin D daily for 6 months and found a decrease in blood pressure of 6.2 mm Hg in the study group, but in the group where plasma vitamin D levels were low at the beginning of the study (<30 ng/ml) the improvement was even better - blood pressure dropped by an average of 7.1 mm Hg (Chen et al. 2014).

Iranian patients with hypertension received vitamin D at a dose of 50,000 IU per week (in those with serum vitamin D levels 20 ng/mL at the start of the research) and 1000 IU per day (in those with 20–30 ng/mL) for 8 weeks (Panahi et al. 2021). This led to an average drop in blood pressure of 5.5 mm Hg. It is interesting to note that even before the patients received the supplement for 8 weeks, the investigators discovered no correlation between serum vitamin D levels and blood pressure.

With the exception of the fact that the vitamin D treatment lasted for 2 months and blood pressure was assessed monthly, Sheikh et al. (2020) also published an investigation on Iranian patients using quite a similar approach. Interestingly, this time the results were inconclusive, and a statistically significant decrease in blood pressure relative to the control group was noted only in the first month and was 6.46 mm Hg, for those supplementing with 1000 IU of vitamin D daily and only 1.65 mm Hg for those taking 50000 IU of vitamin D weekly.

Only in individuals with vitamin D deficiency (<32 ng/ml), according to Larsen et al. (2012), did supplementation with 3000 IU of vitamin D for 20 weeks result in a mean drop in blood pressure of 4 mm Hg.

Arora et al. (2015), Witham et al. (2013), Witham et al. (2014a) and Witham et al. (2014b) found no relationship and the supplementation consisted of:
    - 100000 IU vitamin D every 3 months for 1 year,
    - 100000 IU vitamin D every 2 months for 6 months,
    - 100000 IU vitamin D every 3 months for 1 year,
    - 400 IU (one group) and 4000 IU (other group) vitamin D daily for 6 months, respectively.

What you should know
- Vitamin D has interactions with dozens of different medications.
- Due to the fact that vitamin D is stored in adipose tissue, people with higher BMIs could require higher doses of the vitamin. But be sure to talk to your doctor about how much vitamin D you should be taking.

- In order to support normal bone mineralization, vitamin D maintains sufficient blood calcium and phosphate concentrations.
- In serum, vitamin D has a half-life of roughly 15 days. Without administration via supplementation or dermal synthesis, the amount of vitamin D metabolites would decrease by 50% during this time (Institute of Medicine, Food and Nutrition Board, 2010).
- Blood vitamin D levels below 20 ng/mL (50 nmol/L) are generally regarded as inadequate by health-related organizations (Institute of Medicine, Food and Nutrition Board, 2010).
- Many specialists believe that exposure to the sun for 5 to 30 minutes on the face, arms, hands, and legs at least twice per week, between the hours of 10 a.m. and 4 p.m., is sufficient to produce enough vitamin D (Bouillon, 2017; Holick, 2007; U.S. Department of Health and Human Services, 2014).

References

1. Alpsoy, S., Akyüz, A., Akkoyun, D. C., Gür, D. Ö., Topcu, B., & Tülübas, F. (2016). Vitamin D levels in white coat and sustained hypertension. Blood Pressure Monitoring, 21(3), 131-135.
2. Arora, P., Song, Y., Dusek, J., Plotnikoff, G., Sabatine, M. S., Cheng, S., ... & Wang, T. J. (2015). Vitamin D therapy in individuals with prehypertension or hypertension: the DAYLIGHT trial. Circulation, 131(3), 254-262.
3. Bouillon R. (2017). Comparative analysis of nutritional guidelines for vitamin D. Nature reviews. Endocrinology, 13(8), 466–479. https://doi.org/10.1038/nrendo.2017.31
4. Chen, W. R., Liu, Z. Y., Shi, Y., Wang, H., Sha, Y., & Dai Chen, Y. (2014). Vitamin D and nifedipine in the treatment of Chinese patients with grades I–II essential hypertension: A randomized placebo-controlled trial. Atherosclerosis, 235(1), 102-109.
5. de Paula, T. P., Moreira, J. S., Sperb, L. F., Muller, M. E. P., Steemburgo, T., & Viana, L. V. (2020). Efficacy of single-dose cholecalciferol in the blood pressure of patients with type 2 diabetes, hypertension and hypovitaminoses D. Scientific reports, 10(1), 1-8.
6. Holick M. F. (2007). Vitamin D deficiency. The New England journal of medicine, 357(3), 266–281. https://doi.org/10.1056/NEJMra070553
7. Institute of Medicine, Food and Nutrition Board. Dietary Reference Intakes for Calcium and Vitamin D. Washington, DC: National Academy Press, 2010
8. Larsen, T., Mose, F. H., Bech, J. N., Hansen, A. B., & Pedersen, E. B. (2012). Effect of cholecalciferol supplementation during winter months in

patients with hypertension: a randomized, placebo-controlled trial. American journal of hypertension, 25(11), 1215-1222.

9. Panahi, Y., Namazi, S., Rostami-Yalmeh, J., Sahebi, E., Khalili, N., Jamialahmadi, T., & Sahebkar, A. (2021). Effect of Vitamin D Supplementation on the Regulation of Blood Pressure in Iranian Patients with Essential Hypertension: A Clinical Trial. In Natural Products and Human Diseases (pp. 501-511). Springer, Cham.

10. Sheikh, V., Mozaianimonfared, A., Gharakhani, M., & Poorolajal, J. (2020). Effect of vitamin D supplementation versus placebo on essential hypertension in patients with vitamin D deficiency: a double-blind randomized clinical trial. The Journal of Clinical Hypertension, 22(10), 1867-1873.

11. U.S. Department of Health and Human Services. The Surgeon General's Call to Action to Prevent Skin Cancerexternal link disclaimer. Washington, DC: U.S. Dept of Health and Human Services, Office of the Surgeon General; 2014.

12. Wang, L., Ma, J., Manson, J. E., Buring, J. E., Gaziano, J. M., & Sesso, H. D. (2013). A prospective study of plasma vitamin D metabolites, vitamin D receptor gene polymorphisms, and risk of hypertension in men. European journal of nutrition, 52(7), 1771-1779.

13. Witham, M. D., Price, R. J., Struthers, A. D., Donnan, P. T., Messow, C. M., Ford, I., & McMurdo, M. E. (2013). Cholecalciferol treatment to reduce blood pressure in older patients with isolated systolic hypertension: the VitDISH randomized controlled trial. JAMA internal medicine, 173(18), 1672-1679.

14. Witham, M. D., Ireland, S., Houston, J. G., Gandy, S. J., Waugh, S., MacDonald, T. M., ... & Struthers, A. D. (2014a). Vitamin D therapy to reduce blood pressure and left ventricular hypertrophy in resistant hypertension: randomized, controlled trial. Hypertension, 63(4), 706-712

15. Witham, M. D., Price, R. J., Struthers, A. D., Donnan, P. T., Messow, M., McConnachie, A., ... & McMurdo, M. E. (2014b). Effect of vitamin D supplementation on orthostatic hypotension: data from the vitamin D in isolated systolic hypertension randomized controlled trial. Journal of Hypertension, 32(8), 1693-1699.

1.2.22 Watermelon extract

US researchers evaluated the effects of watermelon extract supplementation on 14 adults (Figueroa et al. 2012). After six weeks, there was an average reduction of 15.1 mm Hg in blood pressure.

> ***Watermelon extract - how was the intervention conducted?***
> L-citrulline/L-arginine (2/1) is present in watermelon extract,

which was given orally at a quantity of 6 grams per day (0.21 oz). The publication's authors estimate that it is roughly similar to 2.3 pounds (1.04 kg) of raw red watermelon.

6 grams per day → 6 weeks → 15.1 mm Hg

What you should know

- Watermelon contains up to 92% water (Naz et al., 2014).
- The tomato, which is known for its high lycopene content, has up to 40% less lycopene than watermelon (U.S. Department of Agriculture website)
- Due to its high glycemic index (GI), watermelon may cause an increase in blood sugar levels.

References

1. Figueroa, A., Sanchez-Gonzalez, M. A., Wong, A., & Arjmandi, B. H. (2012). Watermelon extract supplementation reduces ankle blood pressure and carotid augmentation index in obese adults with prehypertension or hypertension. American journal of hypertension, 25(6), 640-643.
2. Naz, A., Butt, M. S., Sultan, M. T., Qayyum, M. M., & Niaz, R. S. (2014). Watermelon lycopene and allied health claims. EXCLI journal, 13, 650–660.
3. U.S. Department of Agriculture, https://agresearchmag.ars.usda.gov/2002/jun/lyco, accessed: 26th May 2022,

1.2.23 Others

Two of the publications found were difficult to clearly assign to a specific category within supplements. Llopis-González et al. (2015) checked whether there was an association between hypertension and the intake of fat-soluble vitamins A, D and E on almost 700 Spanish subjects. However, no such relationship was found. In turn, Mazza et al. (2019) supplemented Italian participants with a product consisting of red yeast rice, berberine, Coenzyme Q10, folic acid and chrome and found no effect on blood pressure after 3 months. I won't go through the methodology because neither research concluded that the interventions under consideration had a reducing effect on blood pressure.

References

1. Llopis-González, A., Rubio-López, N., Pineda-Alonso, M., Martín-Escudero, J. C., Javier Chaves, F., Redondo, M., & Morales-Suarez-Varela, M. (2015). Hypertension and the fat-soluble vitamins A, D and E. International journal of environmental research and public health, 12(3), 2793-2809.

2. Mazza, A., Schiavon, L., Rigatelli, G., Torin, G., & Lenti, S. (2019). The effects of a new generation of nutraceutical compounds on lipid profile and glycaemia in subjects with pre-hypertension. High Blood Pressure & Cardiovascular Prevention, 26(4), 345-350.

1.2.24 Summary of supplementary interventions - what works

In summary, out of the supplementation publications reviewed, the following appeared to have little effect or the results were inconclusive:

- Folic acid
- Peptides
- Selenium
- Association between hypertension and intake of fat-soluble vitamins A, D and E
- Supplement containing yeast rice, Berberine, Coenzyme Q10, folic acid and chrome.

If a substance, plant, or mixture appears on the list above, it does not automatically prove that it has no effect on hypertension; rather, it simply means that during the study period, no relevant blood pressure-lowering effect had been shown in the population being studied and under the given conditions.

What works? The most effective interventions for high blood pressure included the application of Indian kudzu (blood pressure decreased by 25 mm Hg), *Mellisa officinalis* (blood pressure decreased by 21.45 mm Hg), Quercetin (blood pressure decreased by 19.5 mm Hg), American ginseng (blood pressure decreased by 17.4 mm Hg), and *Orthosiphon stamineus* (blood pressure decreased by 15 mm Hg). Figure 5 displays the specifics of the interventions that have been examined.

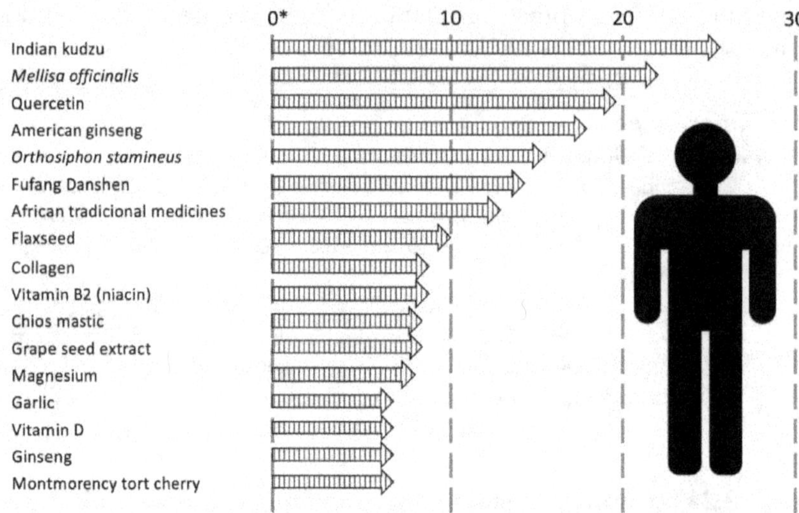

* - blood pressure reduction scale in units of mm Hg, which literally means the average of the highest systolic blood pressure reduction values reported in a given publication

Figure 5. The most effective supplementary interventions that affect blood pressure.

PART 2. PHYSICAL ACTIVITY

The analysis of more than 50 clinical trials led to the creation of this section. These articles combine a variety of approaches, from those that demonstrate conventional aerobic training to varieties of physical activity that are difficult to pinpoint. This section will be divided into the following subsections: aerobic, anaerobic, and combined training. However, this separation is not entirely obvious in many cases, so I have added a summary at the end where I have taken all the publications into account.

Before we move on to the description of the most effective types of physical activity for hypertension, it is worth knowing a few terms that appear in methodologies in publications:

- Aerobic training - a form of activity that involves light to moderate intensity movements performed over an extended length of time with oxygen as the primary energy source. It is believed that aerobic training should meet the following conditions: up to 50% VO2 max in untrained subjects, up to 80% VO2 max in trained subjects, about 50-70% of your maximum heart rate (some sources say it can be up to 80% Max HR).
- Anaerobic training - a type of vigorous activity that is shorter in length than aerobic exercise and in which oxygen is not the body's major source of energy. The main forms of anaerobic exercise include sprinting and strength training.
- Aerobic threshold (AT) - the point at which the body must switch from aerobic to anaerobic metabolism, which differs in energy source. It is more specifically described as the time when the blood's level of lactic acid, a sign of anaerobic metabolism, starts to rise. There are a variety of more or less accurate ways to estimate AT, from laboratory techniques (such as determining the amount of lactic acid in the blood) to simplified techniques based on straightforward mathematics (based on heart rate).

- Borg scale - The Borg Rating of Perceived Exertion (RPE) is a way to measure the level of intensity of physical activity. On this scale of 6 to 20 (a 15-point scale), 6 indicates no exertion (e.g., resting) and 20 indicates maximum exertion. Individual Borg scale indications in further detail:
  - 6 - No exertion at all, relaxed;
  - 7 - Extremely light;
  - 8; 9 - Very light;
  - 10; 11 - Light;
  - 12 - Moderate;
  - 13 - Somewhat hard;
  - 14; 15 - Hard;
  - 16; 17 - Very hard;
  - 18; 19 - Extremely hard;
  - 20 - Maximal exertion.
- Combined training - a type of physical activity that combines elements of aerobic and anaerobic activity.
- max HR- is the highest number of heart beats per minute that your heart can perform during its highest stress. To determine your max HR you can either have it measured by a professional (direct measurement is the most accurate) or you can use a simple formula: 220 minus your age. The result of this equation is not exact but gives you an approximate estimation of your max HR.
- Heart rate reserve (HRR) - the difference between a person's resting heart rate and maximum heart rate. HRR can be calculated using the formula HRR = max HR - rest HR.
- Metabolic equivalents (METs) - the term used to indicate the intensity of an exercise or activity. One MET is the amount of energy your body uses while at rest (in a seated or lying position), while two METs is the amount of energy your body utilizes during an activity. The average amount of oxygen used by the human body at rest is 3.5 ml per kilogram of body weight every minute. For a person weighing 154

pounds (70 kg) this means that the whole body uses an average of 245 ml of oxygen per minute. A correspondingly higher effort raises the average oxygen consumption. Exercises up to 3 METs are considered light (sitting, washing dishes, fishing), between 3-6 METs moderate (golf, brisk walking) and above 6 METs vigorous (cycling, running etc.).

- Respiratory compensation point (RCP) - the point at which the amount of lactic acid in the blood increases rapidly and the excessive excretion of carbon dioxide begins.

- VO2 max - a measurement of an individual's maximum aerobic capacity that takes into account their body's capacity to absorb oxygen while exercising. Around the ages of 18 to 20, this indicator achieves its maximum value. Age-related declines in respiratory and cardiovascular function are the main causes of VO2 max reduction. You can determine your VO2 max in a variety of ways, ranging from extremely accurate laboratory tests to slightly less accurate self-tests. Asking an expert about it or measuring it with tools like digital watches and other fitness equipment that can forecast this parameter are both acceptable choices. Knowing your VO2 max value will definitely allow you to better understand the content of this chapter.

2.1 AEROBIC TRAINING

I have included 32 studies that examined the impact of the following forms of aerobic activity on hypertension in this chapter:

- beach tennis,
- dancing,
- forest trips,
- interval training,
- pilates,
- stair climbing,
- swimming,
- Tai Chi,
- walking (or brisk walking),
- other, not elsewhere classified.

All of the aforementioned activities showed a statistically significant blood pressure-lowering effect; the effect was not always very large, but in this chapter none of the factors were found to be statistically insignificant.

2.1.1 Beach tennis

In a single session of beach tennis, participants from Brazil who were hypertensive had a reduction in blood pressure, according to Carpes et al. (2021). Blood pressure was shown to be lowered on average by 6 mm Hg after only one session. I won't discuss the specifics of the methodology mentioned in that publication.

References

1. Carpes, L., Jacobsen, A., Domingues, L., Jung, N., & Ferrari, R. (2021). Recreational beach tennis reduces 24-h blood pressure in adults with hypertension: a randomized crossover trial. European Journal of Applied Physiology, 121(5), 1327-1336.

2.1.2 Cycling

The effect of cycling has been reported in five publications (Brito et al. 2018, Liang et al. 2021, Pedralli et al. 2020, Santos et al. 2016, Sikiru et al. 2014). Sikiru et al. (2014) reported the most notable blood pressure drop of 13.94 mm Hg in a group of male Nigerian patients with mild to moderate hypertension who trained for 8 weeks on a bicycle ergometer. Three crossover interventions that reduced blood pressure by 7.7-9.4 mm Hg were described by Santos et al. (2016). The patients mentioned by Liang et al. (2021) experienced a mean blood pressure reduction of 9 mm Hg after completing 12 weeks of training on a cycle ergometer. As described by Brito et al. (2018), subjects underwent progressive aerobic training on the cycle ergometer, split between morning and evening sessions. Only after evening training did blood pressure drop on average by 5 to 8 mm Hg after 10 weeks. After 8 weeks of cycle ergometer training, Pedralli et al. (2020) noted an average blood pressure reduction of 5.1 mm Hg.

Cycling - how was the intervention conducted?

Patients from Nigeria who had mild to moderate essential hypertension underwent the 8-week intervention Sikiru et al. (2014) described. They exercised for 45 to 60 minutes three times a week at an intensity of 60 to 79 percent of their HRR. Initial cycling speed was 50 rpm with a workload of 100 kgm (17 watts) and an intensity of 60% of HRR. Within two weeks, this intensity was increased to 79 percent of HRR and remained at this level until the end of the trainings. Training sessions lasted 45 minutes for the first two weeks of the intervention, and subsequently increased to 60 minutes.

A group of 20 Brazilian men undertook three interventions, which Santos et al. (2016) report. During and after each intervention, changes in the men's blood pressure were recorded. Not counting the control intervention, light intensity and moderate intensity 45-minute interventions were also carried out - at an intensity level of 50% and 75% of max HR, which were based on cycling. After 5 hours, there was a reduction in blood pressure of 7.7 mm Hg in the 50% max HR group and 9.4 mm Hg in the group that cycled at 75% max HR intensity.

Five times per week, Chinese patients participated in a 12-week intervention on a moderately intense cycle ergometer. Moderate intensity was determined by the study's authors as corresponding to 75% of the individual maximum metabolic equivalent (MET). The intervention consisted of 3 sessions per round:

- 3-minute warm up (cycling without resistance)
- 45 minutes of cycle exercise at 75% of a maximal metabolic equivalent level (60 rpm)
- 10 minutes of recovery (cycling without resistance).

The total was 58 minutes per day for 5 days per week.

Brazilian men aged 30-65 were the study subjects for a 10-week intervention that occurred three times each week, according to Brito et al. (2018). The duration of each group cycling (cycle ergometer) training session was 30 to 45 minutes, with intensities ranging from the anaerobic threshold (AT) to 10% below the respiratory compensation point. Participants were involved in morning (7-9 a.m.) and evening training sessions (6-8 p.m.). A bachelor's degree holder in physical education supervised all of the classes. Exercise time went from 30 to 45 minutes throughout the first four weeks. Starting with the fifth week, the intensity was raised every two weeks from the anaerobic threshold (AT) heart rate to a heart rate that was 10% below the respiratory compensation point (RCP).

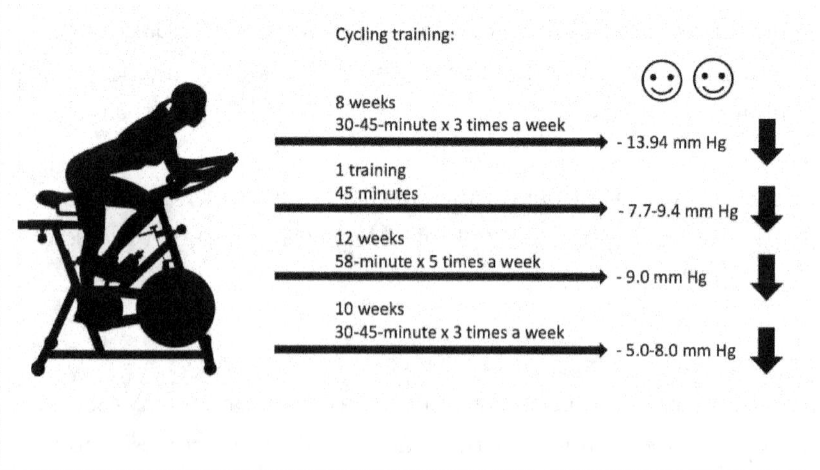

What you should know

- Cycling can be an excellent introduction for those new to exercise because it has health benefits that are experienced even by sedentary persons (Kaya et al. 2018).
- A study indicated that older persons who biked outside had better cognitive health (Leyland et al. 2019)

- Cycling has a beneficial impact on total cholesterol, claims one review. While reducing triglyceride and LDL (bad) cholesterol levels, it may increase HDL (good) cholesterol levels (Chavarrias et al. 2019).

- Low-intensity morning rides can help you lose weight, improve your endurance (Aird et al. 2018).

- In one study, cycling for commuting and recreation was consistently linked to a decreased incidence of type 2 diabetes in Danish adults. Additionally, the findings show a decreased risk of type 2 diabetes with late-life cycling participation (Rasmussen et al. 2016).

- Cycling was linked to at least a 24 percent lower all-cause mortality risk among diabetics when compared to non-cyclists, regardless of other forms of exercise or potential confounders. Comparing consistent non-cyclists to those who started cycling during a 5-year period, there was at least a 35% reduction in the risk of all-cause mortality (Ried-Larsen et al. 2021).

References

1. Aird, T. P., Davies, R. W., & Carson, B. P. (2018). Effects of fasted vs fed-state exercise on performance and post-exercise metabolism: A systematic review and meta-analysis. Scandinavian journal of medicine & science in sports, 28(5), 1476-1493.
2. Brito, L., Pecanha, T., Fecchio, R., Rezende, R., Sousa, P., Silva-Júnior, N., ... & Forjaz, C. (2018). Morning vs evening aerobic training effects on blood pressure in treated hypertension. Medicine & Science in Sports & Exercise, 51(4), 653-662.
3. Chavarrias, M., Carlos-Vivas, J., Collado-Mateo, D., & Pérez-Gómez, J. (2019). Health benefits of indoor cycling: A systematic review. Medicina, 55(8), 452.
4. Kaya, F., Nar, D., & Erzeybek, M. S. (2018). Effect of Spinning Cycling Training on Body Composition in Women. Journal of education and training studies, 6(4), 154-160.
5. Leyland, L. A., Spencer, B., Beale, N., Jones, T., & Van Reekum, C. M. (2019). The effect of cycling on cognitive function and well-being in older adults. PloS one, 14(2), e0211779.
6. Liang, J., Zhang, X., Xia, W., Tong, X., Qiu, Y., Qiu, Y., ... & Tao, J. (2021). Promotion of Aerobic Exercise Induced Angiogenesis Is

Associated With Decline in Blood Pressure in Hypertension: Result of EXCAVATION-CHN1. Hypertension, 77(4), 1141-1153.

7. Pedralli, M. L., Marschner, R. A., Kollet, D. P., Neto, S. G., Eibel, B., Tanaka, H., & Lehnen, A. M. (2020). Different exercise training modalities produce similar endothelial function improvements in individuals with prehypertension or hypertension: A randomized clinical trial. Scientific reports, 10(1), 1-9.

8. Rasmussen, M. G., Grøntved, A., Blond, K., Overvad, K., Tjønneland, A., Jensen, M. K., & Østergaard, L. (2016). Associations between recreational and commuter cycling, changes in cycling, and type 2 diabetes risk: a cohort study of Danish men and women. PLoS medicine, 13(7), e1002076.

9. Ried-Larsen, M., Rasmussen, M. G., Blond, K., Overvad, T. F., Overvad, K., Steindorf, K., ... & Grøntved, A. (2021). Association of cycling with all-cause and cardiovascular disease mortality among persons with diabetes: the European Prospective Investigation Into Cancer and Nutrition (EPIC) Study. JAMA internal medicine, 181(9), 1196-1205.

10. Santos, L. P., Moraes, R. S., Vieira, P. J., Ash, G. I., Waclawovsky, G., Pescatello, L. S., & Umpierre, D. (2016). Effects of aerobic exercise intensity on ambulatory blood pressure and vascular responses in resistant hypertension: a crossover trial. Journal of hypertension, 34(7), 1317-1324.

11. Sikiru, L., & Okoye, G. C. (2014). Therapeutic effect of continuous exercise training program on serum creatinine concentration in men with hypertension: a randomized controlled trial. Ghana medical journal, 48(3), 135-142.

2.1.3 Dancing

Dancing has been shown to lower blood pressure, with reductions ranging from 3.5 to 10.7 mm Hg (Maruf et al. 2016, Kaholokula et al. 2017, 2021). The Hawaiian traditional Hula dance, which is performed by Native Hawaiians and Pacific Islanders who suffer from hypertension, was shown to be the most beneficial (Kaholokula et al. 2017). Hula dance lessons were also shown in a later study of Kaholokula et al. (2021) to lower blood pressure by an average of 3.5 mm Hg in comparison to the control group. In the study by Maruf et al. (2016), which involved Nigerian volunteers over the age of 65, aerobic dance sessions over a period of 12 weeks also had an effect, resulting in a reduction of 7.1 mm Hg.

Dancing - how was the intervention conducted?

Kaholokula et al. (2017) in Honolulu, Hawaii, conducted a study to test a 12-week hula dance-based intervention combined with 3 hours of hypertension self-care education. The physical activity program consisted of the following (two 60-min classes per week):

- 5–15 min - normal range of motion; stretches focusing on legs, arms, lower back; low-level, aerobic activity at 25–40 % MPHR (according to the authors: maximum predicted heart rate, this can be considered equivalent to max HR mentioned above)
- 20–40 min - 40–85 % VO2 max or 50–70 % MPHR; between 12 and 16 on the Borg scale (these parameters are described above);
- 3–10 min - low-level, aerobic activity.

It's important to keep in mind that the hula dance lessons mentioned above were led by a professional hula dancer.

120 newly diagnosed individuals with mild to moderate hypertension underwent a 12-week intervention by Maruf et al. (2016) that included an instructor-led class using a 45-minute fitness dance video disc. Classes were held three times a week, at a maximum heart rate of 50%–70%. Participants watched the same dance video disc every time, and an instructor was present each time. The physical activity program included:

- 5 min. - warm-up - stretching exercises for the arms, legs, and torso
- 35 min. - bouncing movement on the leg, forward and backward movement, jumping, shoulder movements, arm stretching, trunk stretching, rolling and bending of the trunk, hip twisting, and chest movement
- 5 min. - cooldown phase - stretching exercises for the arms, legs, and torso, as during the warm-up phase

Although Kaholokula et al. (2021)'s result (mean reduction of 3.5 mm Hg) was not especially notable, it is a follow-up to Kaholokula et al (2017). This time, the intervention lasted for six months and included more people. Although participants' blood pressure dropped as much as 15.3 mm Hg, the control group also had drops as high as 11.8 mm Hg. Only 3.5 mm Hg separated the study group from the control group, where only the educational intervention was implemented.

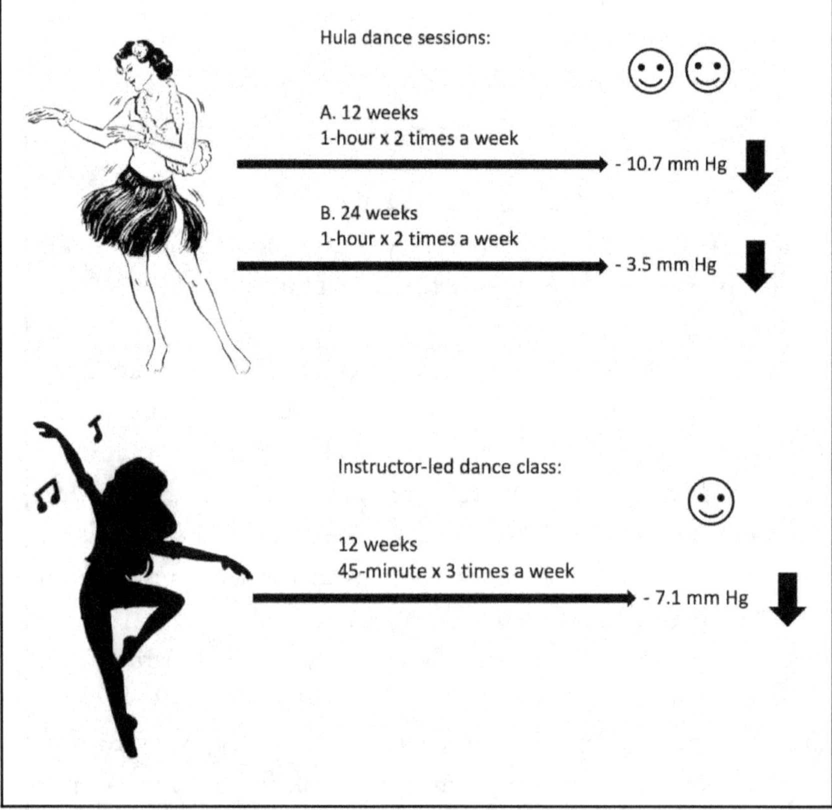

What you should know

- Dancing is a great way to increase physical fitness and social skills, which will improve mental health (Bremer 2007).

- Even moderate physical activity can boost metabolism in parts of the brain that are crucial for learning and memory (Dougherty et al. 2017).

- Participating in recreational activities is linked to a lower incidence of dementia (Verghese et al. 2003).

- More so than walking, moderate-intensity dancing was linked to a lower risk of mortality from cardiovascular disease (Merom et al. 2016).

- Dancing can help older adults considerably increase their aerobic capacity, lower body muscle endurance, strength, and flexibility, as well as their balance, agility, and gait. Additionally, dancing may increase the lower body's bone and muscle mass in this group, minimize their risk of falls, and improve their cardiovascular health (Keogh et al. 2009).

References

1. Bremer, Z. (2007). Dance as a form of exercise. British Journal of General Practice, 57(535), 166-166.
2. Dougherty, R. J., Schultz, S. A., Kirby, T. K., Boots, E. A., Oh, J. M., Edwards, D., ... & Okonkwo, O. C. (2017). Moderate physical activity is associated with cerebral glucose metabolism in adults at risk for Alzheimer's disease. Journal of Alzheimer's Disease, 58(4), 1089-1097.
3. Kaholokula, J. K. A., Look, M., Mabellos, T., Ahn, H. J., Choi, S. Y., Sinclair, K. I. A., ... & de Silva, M. (2021). A cultural dance program improves hypertension control and cardiovascular disease risk in Native Hawaiians: A randomized controlled trial. Annals of Behavioral Medicine, 55(10), 1006-1018.
4. Kaholokula, J. K. A., Look, M., Mabellos, T., Zhang, G., de Silva, M., Yoshimura, S., ... & Sinclair, K. I. A. (2017). Cultural dance program improves hypertension management for Native Hawaiians and Pacific Islanders: a pilot randomized trial. Journal of racial and ethnic health disparities, 4(1), 35-46.
5. Keogh, J. W., Kilding, A., Pidgeon, P., Ashley, L., & Gillis, D. (2009). Physical benefits of dancing for healthy older adults: a review. Journal of aging and physical activity, 17(4), 479-500.
6. Maruf, F. A., Akinpelu, A. O., Salako, B. L., & Akinyemi, J. O. (2016). Effects of aerobic dance training on blood pressure in individuals with uncontrolled hypertension on two antihypertensive drugs: a randomized clinical trial. Journal of the American Society of Hypertension, 10(4), 336-345.

7. Merom, D., Ding, D., & Stamatakis, E. (2016). Dancing participation and cardiovascular disease mortality: a pooled analysis of 11 population-based British cohorts. American journal of preventive medicine, 50(6), 756-760.

8. Verghese, J., Lipton, R. B., Katz, M. J., Hall, C. B., Derby, C. A., Kuslansky, G., ... & Buschke, H. (2003). Leisure activities and the risk of dementia in the elderly. New England Journal of Medicine, 348(25), 2508-2516.

2.1.4 Forest trip

In a study conducted by Mao et al. (2012), Chinese men between the ages of 60 and 75 were exposed to broad-leaved evergreens for seven days. Although the graph indicates that the effect was statistically significant but not particularly large (a reduction of about 4 mm Hg), the report does not specify the precise number by which blood pressure was decreased. I won't go into detail about this intervention's specifics due to the small effect.

References

1. Mao, G. X., Cao, Y. B., Lan, X. G., He, Z. H., Chen, Z. M., Wang, Y. Z., ... & Yan, J. (2012). Therapeutic effect of forest bathing on human hypertension in the elderly. Journal of cardiology, 60(6), 495-502.

2.1.5 Interval training

The study by Lamina (2012) indicated that 8 weeks of interval training at intensities between 60 and 79 percent of max HR could lower blood pressure by as much as 15.7 mm Hg in Nigerian participants.

Interval training - how was the intervention conducted?

For eight weeks, participants in this study went to exercise sessions three times a week. In one session, it was as follows:

- 10-minutes - warm up - pedaling at zero resistance

- 45-minutes - the group exercised on a cycle ergometer at a moderate intensity of 60-79% max HR; the initial workload was 100 kgm (17 watts) and was increased at a pedaling speed of 50 rpm to reach 60% HR reserve, which then increased during the first two weeks to 79% HR reserve and this value was maintained for the remainder of the training period in a 1:1 ratio of 6 minutes each. During the 6 min rest interval period, participants cycled at zero intensity. Two weeks later, this stage was extended from 45 minutes to 60 minutes and another 10-minute cool down was established by pedaling at zero resistance.

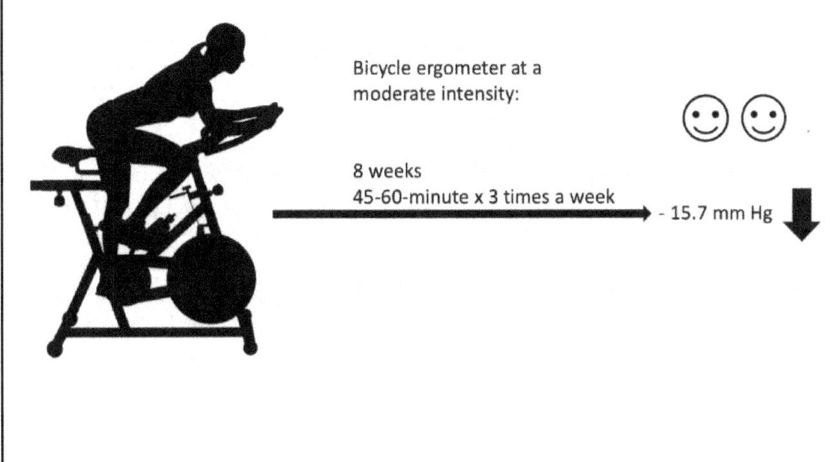

What you should know

- Researchers compared the number of calories burned during 30 minutes of running, biking, weight training, and interval training and discovered that compared to other forms of exercise, interval training burnt 25–30% more calories (Falcone et al. 2015).
- High-intensity interval training has been shown to cause a variety of physiological changes that enhance exercise capacity, including maximal oxygen uptake, aerobic endurance, anaerobic capacity (Atakan et al. 2021).

- High-intensity interval training showed improvements in insulin sensitivity, blood lipid levels, body fat percentage, and cardiovascular fitness (Fisher et al. 2015).

References

1. Atakan, M. M., Li, Y., Koşar, Ş. N., Turnagöl, H. H., & Yan, X. (2021). Evidence-based effects of high-intensity interval training on exercise capacity and health: a review with historical perspective. International journal of environmental research and public health, 18(13), 7201.
2. Falcone, P. H., Tai, C. Y., Carson, L. R., Joy, J. M., Mosman, M. M., McCann, T. R., ... & Moon, J. R. (2015). Caloric expenditure of aerobic, resistance, or combined high-intensity interval training using a hydraulic resistance system in healthy men. The Journal of Strength & Conditioning Research, 29(3), 779-785.
3. Fisher, G., Brown, A. W., Bohan Brown, M. M., Alcorn, A., Noles, C., Winwood, L., ... & Allison, D. B. (2015). High intensity interval-vs moderate intensity-training for improving cardiometabolic health in overweight or obese males: a randomized controlled trial. PloS one, 10(10), e0138853.
4. Lamina, S. (2012). Effect of interval exercise training programme on C-reactive protein in the non-pharmacological management of hypertension: a randomized controlled trial. African Journal of Medicine and Medical Sciences, 41(4), 379-386.

2.1.6 Pilates

Twelve volunteers, ranging in age from 44 to 66, were evaluated by Rocha et al. (2020) to determine the impact of a single Pilates session on blood pressure. Blood pressure measurements taken up to an hour after the exercise decreased by 7.4 mm Hg on average.

Pilates - how was the intervention conducted?

The single Pilates session described in the publication consisted of the following steps:

- 8-10 minutes - warm-up including stretching and upper and lower body calisthenics
- approximately 50 minutes - each of the following exercises

---

were performed in 10 repetitions:
  o squat (Swiss ball)
  o shoulder adduction (reformer)
  o knee extension (reformer)
  o seated rowing (cadillac)
  o hip extension (wall unit)
  o unilateral shoulder adduction (wall unit)
  o knee extension (cadillac)
  o unilateral hip adduction (cadillac)
  o shoulder extension (reformer)
  o hip extension ('bridge')
  o shoulder flection (reformer)
  o unilateral hip adduction (cadillac)
  o trunk extension (barrel)
  o hip extension (step chair)
  o elbow extension (wall unit)
  o sit-ups

The publication includes pictures of each exercise - you can see what they look like.

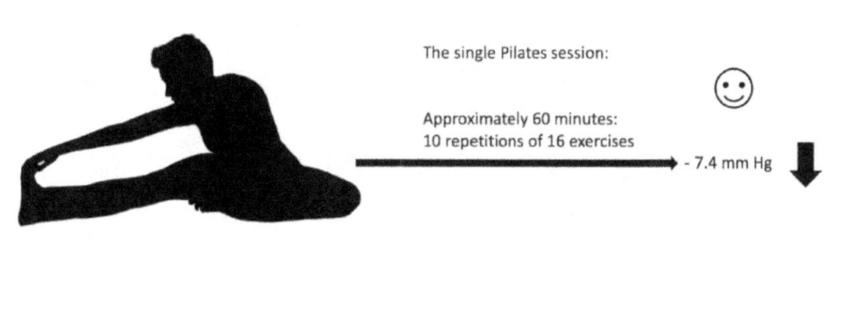

What you should know

- Pilates enhances quality of life by positively affecting depression and pain, particularly back pain (Eliks et al. 2019).
- The pilates method could be an effective form of rehabilitation that can enhance general health, sports

performance, and aid in the avoidance and easing of injuries and musculoskeletal system diseases (Cruz et al. 2016).

- Pilates exercises are a therapeutic method that effectively, safely, and non-invasively reduce menstrual pain (Khadiga et al. 2019).

References

1. Cruz, J. C., Liberali, R., Cruz, T. M. F. D., & Netto, M. I. A. (2016). The Pilates method in the rehabilitation of musculoskeletal disorders: a systematic review. Fisioterapia em Movimento, 29, 609-622.
2. Eliks, M., Zgorzalewicz-Stachowiak, M., & Zeńczak-Praga, K. (2019). Application of Pilates-based exercises in the treatment of chronic non-specific low back pain: state of the art. Postgraduate medical journal, 95(1119), 41-45.
3. Khadiga, S., Eman, M., Mohamad, F., & Asmaa, M. (2019). Effect of Pilates Exercise on Primary Dysmenorrhea. The Medical Journal of Cairo University, 87(March), 1187-1192.
4. Rocha, J., Cunha, F. A., Cordeiro, R., Monteiro, W., Pescatello, L. S., & Farinatti, P. (2020). Acute effect of a single session of pilates on blood pressure and cardiac autonomic control in middle-aged adults with hypertension. The Journal of Strength & Conditioning Research, 34(1), 114-123.

2.1.7 Stair climbing

In the study described by Wong et al. (2018), Korean participants underwent a 12-week intervention that involved climbing 192 steps 2–5 times each day for 4 days per week. After this time, a 6 mm Hg average drop in blood pressure was seen. Since this effect was not large I will not describe the details.

References

1. Wong, A., Figueroa, A., Son, W. M., Chernykh, O., & Park, S. Y. (2018). The effects of stair climbing on arterial stiffness, blood pressure, and leg strength in postmenopausal women with stage 2 hypertension. Menopause, 25(7), 731-737.

2.1.8 Swimming (and aquatic exercises)

In all five studies on swimming and water exercise, the effects of such activity on decreasing blood pressure were statistically significant. This effect was not large in the trials reported by Mohr et al. (2014) and Cunha et al. (2018); the reduction was 4-6 mm Hg. The greatest impact was reported by Guimaraes et al. (2018), who found that water-based activities reduced participants' blood pressure by an average of 19.5 mm Hg in Brazil. Guimraes et al. (2013) also reported a notable outcome in which individuals engaged in hot water-based fitness training three times per week for two weeks, with the blood pressure of the subjects dropping by an average of up to 18 mm Hg. After a 20-week intervention, the researchers of the study Wong et al. (2019) reported a 9 mm Hg decrease in blood pressure in women.

Swimming (and aquatic exercises) - how was the intervention conducted?

Patients with resistant hypertension participated in 36 sessions (60 minutes) in a heated pool (32°C [89.6°F]) 3 times per week for 12 weeks (Guimaraes et al. 2018). Each session consisted of the following steps:

- warming up,
- callisthenic exercises,
- walking between 11 to 13 on the Borg scale
- cooling down.

During the experiment, participants were to maintain their usual diet.

In publication of Guimraes et al. (2013), participants also performed heated water-based exercises, this time over a 2-week period. Each session took place in the afternoon (1:30-2:30 p.m.) in a heated water pool (30-32°C). Patients were immersed in warm water up to the xiphoid process level. Sessions lasted 60 minutes and consisted of the following steps:

- 5 min of warming up,
- 20 min of calisthenics (upper and lower limbs),
- 30 min of walking (HR between the anaerobic threshold and respiratory compensation point, 68-85%, respectively, and the Borg scale between 11 and 13)
- 5 min of cooling down and stretching.

One hundred older women (average age, 74) took part in a 20-week swimming training program that combined freestyle, breast stroke, and back stroke as part of the study described by Wong et al. (2019). Classes were held with an instructor.

First five weeks:

- Swimming 25-30 minutes per day 3-4 times per week at low intensity (60% of max HR)

For the next fifteen weeks:

- Swimming 40-45 minutes per day at a moderate intensity of 70% to 75% of the max HR

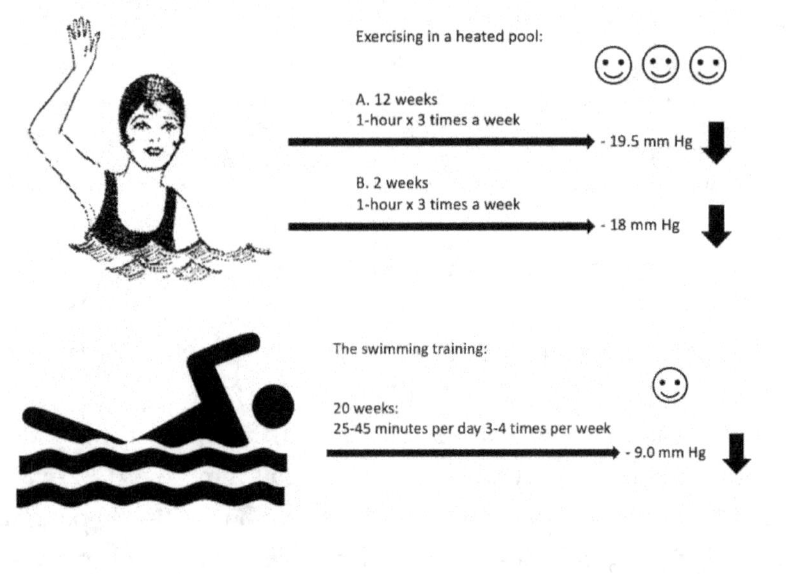

What you should know

- Compared to inactive people, swimmers have around half the risk of death (Centers for Disease Control and Prevention, 2022).
- For inactive, middle-aged, slightly hypertensive women, swimming is an efficient and effective training method for enhancing insulin sensitivity and glucose control (Connolly et al. 2016).
- Exercise in the water can help arthritis sufferers better use their arthritic joints without making their symptoms worse. Rheumatoid arthritis patients who engage in hydrotherapy—exercising in warm water—show greater health gains than those who engage in other activities. Exercise in the water can help lessen osteoarthritis discomfort and increase the usage of injured joints (Centers for Disease Control and Prevention, 2022).

References

1. Centers for Disease Control and Prevention. Health Benefits of Swimming | Healthy Swimming | Healthy Water | CDC. (2022, February 18). Health Benefits of Swimming | Healthy Swimming | Healthy Water | CDC. https://www.cdc.gov/healthywater/swimming/swimmers/health_benefits_water_exercise.html

2. Connolly, L. J., Nordsborg, N. B., Nyberg, M., Weihe, P., Krustrup, P., & Mohr, M. (2016). Low-volume high-intensity swim training is superior to high-volume low-intensity training in relation to insulin sensitivity and glucose control in inactive middle-aged women. European journal of applied physiology, 116(10), 1889-1897.

3. Cunha, R. M., Costa, A. M., Silva, C. N. F., Póvoa, T. I. R., Pescatello, L. S., & Lehnen, A. M. (2018). Postexercise hypotension after aquatic exercise in older women with hypertension: A randomized crossover clinical trial. American Journal of Hypertension, 31(2), 247-252.

4. Guimãraes, G. V., Cruz, L. G., Tavares, A. C., Dorea, E. L., Fernandes-Silva, M. M., & Bocchi, E. A. (2013). Effects of short-term heated water-based exercise training on systemic blood pressure in patients with resistant hypertension: a pilot study. Blood Pressure Monitoring, 18(6), 342-345.

5. Guimãraes, G. V., Fernandes-Silva, M. M., Drager, L. F., de Barros Cruz, L. G., Castro, R. E., Ciolac, E. G., & Bocchi, E. A. (2018). Hypotensive effect of heated water-based exercise persists after 12-week cessation of

training in patients with resistant hypertension. Canadian journal of cardiology, 34(12), 1641-1647.

6. Mohr, M., Nordsborg, N. B., Lindenskov, A., Steinholm, H., Nielsen, H. P., Mortensen, J., ... & Krustrup, P. (2014). High-intensity intermittent swimming improves cardiovascular health status for women with mild hypertension. BioMed research international, 2014.

7. Wong, A., Kwak, Y. S., Scott, S. D., Pekas, E. J., Son, W. M., Kim, J. S., & Park, S. Y. (2019). The effects of swimming training on arterial function, muscular strength, and cardiorespiratory capacity in postmenopausal women with stage 2 hypertension. Menopause, 26(6), 653-658.

2.1.9 Tai Chi

Tai Chi training, which entails slow, fluid movements and deep breaths to calm the exerciser, was the subject of six publications. Blood pressure decreases ranging from 4.27 to 13.33 mm Hg were found to be statistically significant in every experiment. Wen et al. (2021), who combined Wu-style Tai Chi training with traditional Tai Chi training, observed the best results, with a drop in blood pressure of 13.33 mm Hg in individuals with hypertension and hyperlipidemia after six months. In the intervention described by Shou et al. (2019), participants with grade 1 hypertension were subjected to a 24-Style Simplified Tai Chi exercise over the course of three months, and a similarly good result (reduction of 12.74 mm Hg) was obtained. Sun et al. (2015) discussed the results of Tai Chi training that lasted up to 12 months. The average blood pressure of the Chinese participants dropped by 10.43 mm Hg. In a different study, participants in the Tai Chi group took a 3-month course in the 24-form Yang Style Tai Chi, which led to a post-intervention blood pressure drop of 10.28 mm Hg (Chan et al. 2018). After 8 weeks of training, the Yang-style Tai Chi exercise program described by Lo et al. (2012) decreased blood pressure by an average of 7.34 mm Hg. Ma et al. (2018) found the smallest impact when Chinese people 60 years of age and older participated in a simplified 24-form Tai Chi 24-week program. It was discovered that they lowered their blood pressure on average by 4.27 mm Hg.

Tai Chi - how was the intervention conducted?

In the Wen et al. (2021) study, participants were split into two groups: the Wu-style Tai Chi group and the simplified Tai Chi group. For six months, both groups had training three times each week. A Tai Chi Daoyin master with more than 30 years of teaching expertise conducted the 60-minute Wu-style Tai Chi sessions. The instructor gave the students information on the method and the theory underlying Tai Chi Daoyin during the first class. Participants in the subsequent sessions performed 60 forms from the traditional Wu style of Tai Chi and Daoyin for the treatment of cardiovascular diseases. Each session consisted of a warm-up and self-massage, followed by a review of principles, movements, breathing techniques, and relaxation in Wu-style Tai Chi. Additionally, participants were required to spend at least 30 minutes every day practicing Wu-style Tai Chi at home. Each 60-minute simplified Tai Chi group class was led by a professional with 30 years of Tai Chi Daoyin experience, and participants were also urged to practice at home for at least 30 minutes each day. Both groups showed excellent outcomes after six months, albeit the Wu-style Tai Chi practice group's blood pressure decrease was 5.8 mm Hg more than the simplified Tai Chi practice group's.

In a three-month study, participants with grade 1 hypertension underwent simplified Tai Chi exercises once to twice a day (Shou et al. 2019). Participants went through a two-week course with professional rehabilitative therapists to learn the 24-Style Simplified Tai Chi before the actual experiment started. The target heart rate (HR) was set at between 70 and 80 percent of the max HR. The first 10-15 minutes of each session were spent by participants walking or engaging in conditioning exercises. Then, over the period of 20–30 minutes, 2-4 rounds of 24-Style Tai Chi were performed. If the target HR was obtained within 20 to 30 minutes

---

and returned to normal within 5 to 10 minutes following exercise, the training intensity was deemed to be correct. Acceptable exercise intensity was defined as the participant not feeling uncomfortable or out of breath. The exercises were done by the participants in their free time each morning and evening.

Participants in the research conducted by Sun et al. (2015) were older Chinese adults who had hypertension. They were required to practice Tai Chi for a period of one year, attending three hours of group classes per week led by an experienced instructor while also performing two hours of exercise at home at their own pace. Meditation skills, such as breathing, balance, flexibility, focus, soothing, and stress-reduction strategies, were taught to participants in group classes. Participants also used these techniques. One session lasted 90 minutes, followed by a break of 30 minutes (probably in the middle of the session). Unfortunately, several aspects of the process are lacking the necessary specifics.

In the study that was presented by Chan et al. (2018), participants from Hong Kong took part in 24-form Yang Style Tai Chi courses that lasted for one hour and two times a week for a period of three months. Every class was instructed by the same knowledgeable Tai Chi Master who had years of experience. Participants were also requested to perform their own Tai Chi training at home for a minimum of five days per week, lasting a total of thirty minutes per day.

Residents of Taiwan took part in a Yang-style Tai Chi training program that lasted for eight weeks and consisted of three sessions each week lasting an hour each (Lo et al. 2012). The session was divided into three distinct parts:
- 15 minutes: warm-up,
- 40 minutes: Tai Chi exercise session,

- 5 minutes: cool-down.

The training, similar to that described in previous publications, was directed by a knowledgeable instructor. Each movement was repeated at least 6 times.

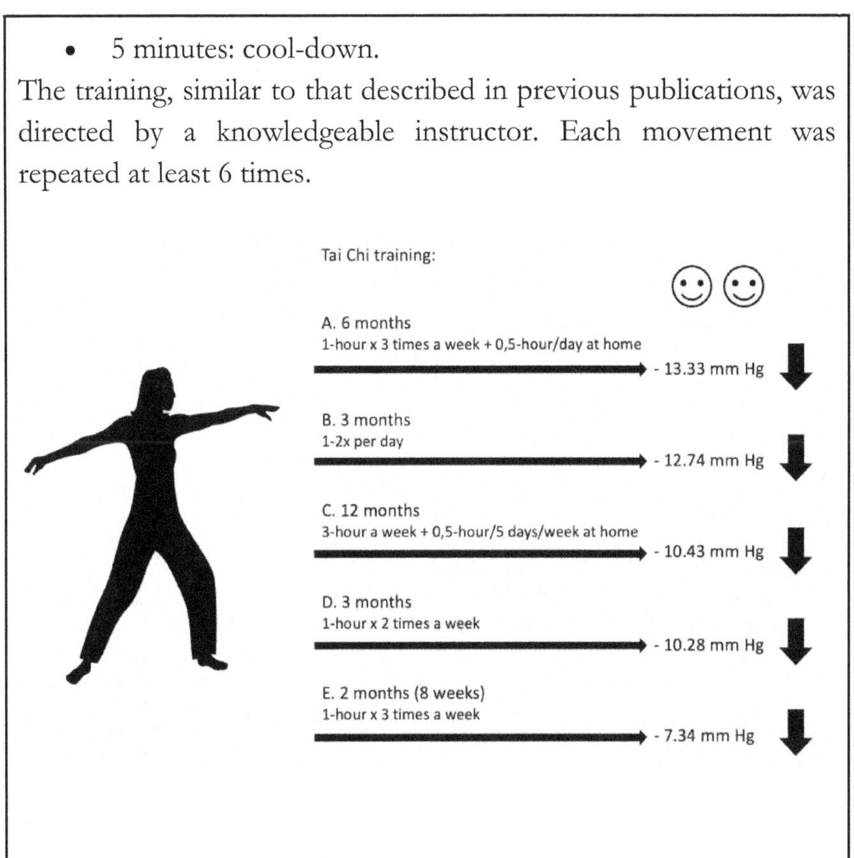

What you should know

- When it comes to reaping the benefits of Tai Chi, experts agree that the best time to start is before you are diagnosed with a chronic condition or experience any functional restrictions. The practice of Tai Chi is extremely risk-free, and its practitioners don't require any specialized gear to get started (Centers for Disease Control and Prevention, 2022).
- Both Qigong and Tai Chi have been found to have beneficial effects on psychological well-being and to reduce symptoms of anxiety and depression in clinical investigations, including randomized controlled trials and meta-analyses (Yeung et al. 2018).

- There is evidence that Tai Chi has the ability to improve cognitive performance in people of advanced age, particularly in the area of executive functioning (Wayne et al. 2014).
- Those who participated in the Tai Chi classes saw significant improvements in the quality of sleep they were able to achieve in comparison to those who were in the control group. Decreased anxiety symptoms were also reported among this group (Caldwell et al. 2016).
- Tai Chi, when done on a regular basis, can be compared to other forms of exercise such as resistance training and brisk walking (Centers for Disease Control and Prevention, 2022).

References

1. Caldwell, K. L., Bergman, S. M., Collier, S. R., Triplett, N. T., Quin, R., Bergquist, J., & Pieper, C. F. (2016). Effects of tai chi chuan on anxiety and sleep quality in young adults: lessons from a randomized controlled feasibility study. Nature and science of sleep, 8, 305.
2. Centers for Disease Control and Prevention. (Health Benefits of Swimming | Healthy Swimming | Healthy Water | CDC. (2022, February 18). Health Benefits of Swimming | Healthy Swimming | Healthy Water | CDC. https://www.cdc.gov/healthywater/swimming/swimmers/health_benefits_water_exercise.html
3. Chan, A. W. K., Chair, S. Y., Lee, D. T. F., Leung, D. Y. P., Sit, J. W. H., Cheng, H. Y., & Taylor-Piliae, R. E. (2018). Tai Chi exercise is more effective than brisk walking in reducing cardiovascular disease risk factors among adults with hypertension: a randomised controlled trial. International journal of nursing studies, 88, 44-52.
4. Lo, H. M., Yeh, C. Y., Chang, S. C., Sung, H. C., & Smith, G. D. (2012). AT ai C hi exercise programme improved exercise behaviour and reduced blood pressure in outpatients with hypertension. International journal of nursing practice, 18(6), 545-551.
5. Ma, C., Zhou, W., Tang, Q., & Huang, S. (2018). The impact of group-based Tai chi on health-status outcomes among community-dwelling older adults with hypertension. Heart & Lung, 47(4), 337-344.
6. Shou, X. L., Wang, L., Jin, X. Q., Zhu, L. Y., Ren, A. H., & Wang, Q. N. (2019). Effect of T'ai Chi exercise on hypertension in young and middle-aged in-service staff. The Journal of Alternative and Complementary Medicine, 25(1), 73-78.
7. Sun, J., & Buys, N. (2015). Community-based mind–body meditative tai chi program and its effects on improvement of blood pressure, weight, renal function, serum lipoprotein, and quality of life in Chinese adults

with hypertension. The American journal of cardiology, 116(7), 1076-1081.

8. Wayne, P. M., Walsh, J. N., Taylor-Piliae, R. E., Wells, R. E., Papp, K. V., Donovan, N. J., & Yeh, G. Y. (2014). Effect of Tai Chi on cognitive performance in older adults: Systematic review and meta-Analysis. Journal of the American Geriatrics Society, 62(1), 25-39.

9. Wen, J., & Su, M. (2021). A randomized trial of Tai Chi on preventing hypertension and hyperlipidemia in middle-aged and elderly patients. International journal of environmental research and public health, 18(10), 5480.

10. Yeung, A., Chan, J. S., Cheung, J. C., & Zou, L. (2018). Qigong and Tai-Chi for mood regulation. Focus, 16(1), 40-47.

2.1.10 Treadmill running

Running on a treadmill has been the subject of research presented in three different papers (Caminiti et al. 2021, Dimeo et al. 2012, Pires et al. 2020). An experiment with 20 participants tested a single session on a treadmill, with half of the participants having hypertension that is resistant to treatment and the other half having hypertension that is not resistant to treatment (Pires et al. 2020). This intervention led to a decrease in blood pressure that ranged from 15.4 to 18.0 mm Hg, and the magnitude of this change was dependent on the amount of time that had passed since the workout. Caminiti et al. (2021) stated that a 12-week intervention resulted in a blood pressure decrease of 3.2-6.9 mm Hg, and Dimeo et al. (2012) reported that a blood pressure drop of 6 mm Hg occurred after 8-12 weeks of training.

Treadmill running - how was the intervention conducted?
Pires et al. (2020) published an article in which the authors described the effect of a single session of aerobic training. The workout consisted of 45 minutes of running on a treadmill at max HR that was between 50-60%. The publication does not provide some of the other specific details of this intervention.

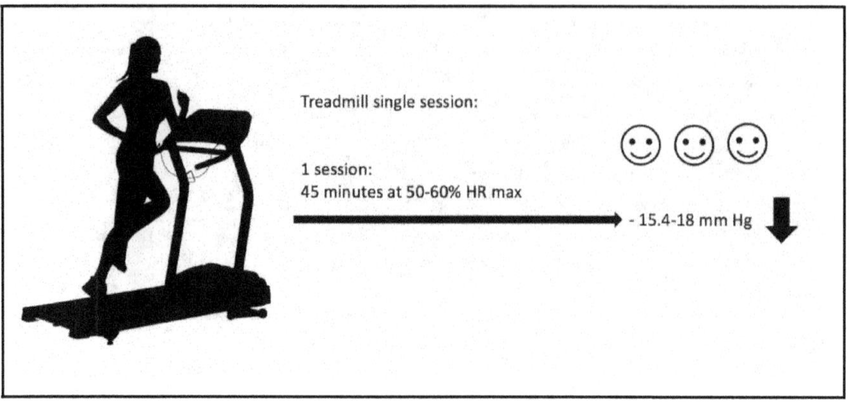

What you should know

- Running, in any of its many forms, can bring a number of health benefits, including a lower risk of depression and anxiety, lower blood pressure, and lower cholesterol and blood sugar levels (Nystoriak and Bhatnagar 2018).

- Walking at a quick pace on a treadmill for ten weeks enhanced the quality of life of female patients diagnosed with group 1 pulmonary hypertension, according to patient reports (Chan et al. 2013).

- Treadmill walking exercise training is an effective treatment program that improves bone mineral status and regulates inflammatory cytokines and blood lipids profile in obese asthmatic patients who have been taking corticosteroids for a long period of time (Abd El-Kader et al. 2016).

- To preserve leg muscle mass, strength, and endurance, treadmill training is a crucial complementary exercise countermeasure (Schneider et al. 2016).

- Before starting any new exercise routine, you should talk to your doctor.

References

1. Abd El-Kader, S. M., Al-Jiffri, O. H., Ashmawy, E. M., & Gaowgzeh, R. A. M. (2016). Treadmill walking exercise modulates bone mineral status and inflammatory cytokines in obese asthmatic patients with long term intake of corticosteroids. African Health Sciences, 16(3), 798-808.

2. Caminiti, G., Iellamo, F., Mancuso, A., Cerrito, A., Montano, M., Manzi, V., & Volterrani, M. (2021). Effects of 12 weeks of aerobic versus combined aerobic plus resistance exercise training on short-term blood pressure variability in patients with hypertension. Journal of Applied Physiology, 130(4), 1085-1092.

3. Chan, L., Chin, L. M., Kennedy, M., Woolstenhulme, J. G., Nathan, S. D., Weinstein, A. A., ... & Keyser, R. E. (2013). Benefits of intensive treadmill exercise training on cardiorespiratory function and quality of life in patients with pulmonary hypertension. Chest, 143(2), 333-343.

4. Dimeo, F., Pagonas, N., Seibert, F., Arndt, R., Zidek, W., & Westhoff, T. H. (2012). Aerobic exercise reduces blood pressure in resistant hypertension. Hypertension, 60(3), 653-658.

5. Nystoriak, M. A., & Bhatnagar, A. (2018). Cardiovascular effects and benefits of exercise. Frontiers in cardiovascular medicine, 5, 135.

6. Pires, N. F., Coelho-Júnior, H. J., Gambassi, B. B., de Faria, A. P. C., Ritter, A. M. V., de Andrade Barboza, C., ... & Júnior, H. M. (2020). Combined aerobic and resistance exercises evokes longer reductions on ambulatory blood pressure in resistant hypertension: a randomized crossover trial. Cardiovascular therapeutics, 2020.

7. Schneider, S. M., Lee, S. M., Feiveson, A. H., Watenpaugh, D. E., Macias, B. R., & Hargens, A. R. (2016). Treadmill exercise within lower body negative pressure protects leg lean tissue mass and extensor strength and endurance during bed rest. Physiological reports, 4(15), e12892.

2.1.11 Other aerobic activity

This chapter includes other publications that describe the effects of aerobic training and could not easily be placed in any of the other sections. It's hard to compare them because they use different methods. The results that were achieved from the various types of aerobic exercise are not very impressive; however, out of the five publications that were reviewed, reductions in blood pressure that were statistically significant were obtained in four of them. After participating in a 12-week aerobic exercise training program, Lopes et al. (2021) observed a reduction in blood pressure ranging from 7.1-10 mm Hg. Similarly, Pagonas et al. (2017) found similar impact after the intervention had been carried out for the same amount of time (i.e., a reduction of 4.9-10 mm Hg). In the study that was conducted and published by Gorostegi-Anduaga et al. (2018), the authors found that the effect of combining various aerobic exercise programs with a dietary intervention for a period of 16 weeks resulted in a reduction in blood pressure that ranged from 4.6 to 8.5 mm Hg on average. In relation, the trial that was carried out by MartinezAguirre-Betolaza et al. (2020) showed that using the same methods led to a decrease in blood pressure that ranged from 4.2 to 6.4 mm Hg. However, Barcellos et al. (2018) in the most recent paper that was analyzed found that after 16 weeks of aerobic exercise, there was no statistically significant influence on the participants' blood pressure.

> ### *Other aerobic activity - how was the intervention conducted?*
> The adoption of an aerobic exercise training program that lasted for 12 weeks and had a moderate intensity was described by Lopes et al. (2021). Training sessions with a supervisor were held three times a week for the participants. Each session included:
> - 10-minute - warmup,
> - 40 minutes - cycling and/or walking at 50% to 70% of VO2 max (11 to 14 on the Borg scale),
> - 10-minute cooldown.
>
> The participants began their first week of training with 20 minutes of exercise at 50% of their VO2 max. From there, the training was prolonged by 5 minutes each week and the intensity was increased by 5% of their VO2 max until they reached 40 minutes of exercise at 70% of their VO2 max.
>
> In the study that was published by Pagonas et al. (2017), the researchers used a methodology in which individuals from Germany took part in a 12-week intervention for 3-5 sessions lasting 30 minutes each. The researchers who were responsible for the approach described the training as exercise that was "pretty hard but still enabled a conversation." This intensity level matched to levels 12-13 on the Borg scale. The training was of a moderate intensity. The sports of walking, jogging, cycling, and swimming were suggested as excellent first choices. The participants were not

required to follow a predetermined exercise routine, nor were they guided through any of the exercises by a trained expert.

The research conducted by Gorostegi-Anduaga et al. (2018) included 175 Hispanic volunteers who were either overweight or obese and had hypertension. The subjects were separated into the following groups, each receiving a different kind of training:

- HV-MICT group - continuous training at high volume and moderate intensity for 45 minutes (65% VO2peak)
- HV-HIIT group - high volume, high intensity interval training (one day on treadmill 4x4 min at 90% VO2peak and 29 min at 65% VO2peak and one day on exercise bike 18x30 s at 90% VO2peak and 36 min at 65% VO2peak)
- LV-HIIT group - low volume, high intensity interval training (one day on the treadmill 2x4 min at 90% VO2peak and 12 min at 65% VO2peak).

The training lasted for a total of 16 weeks and consisted of twice weekly sessions led by an experienced instructor. The intensity of the workout was modified according to each person's HRR and perceived exertion index (6-20 Borg points). The warm-up for each session lasted between five and ten minutes, while the cooldown lasted ten minutes. One of the most important aspects of each session consisted of performing a variety of cardiovascular activities, which included running on a treadmill on one day of the week and riding a bike on another day. Different groups completed their workouts for a different amount of time; the HV-MICT and HV-HIIT groups worked out for a total of 45 minutes, while the LV-HIIT group worked out for a total of 20 minutes. Every participant adhered to a low-calorie, sodium-restricted diet that ranged from 3-6 grams per day (0.11-0.21 oz). The goal of the diet was to deliver 25% fewer calories than the average daily energy expenditure. This diet was comparable to the DASH diet in that it had 15% protein, 55% carbohydrates, and 30% fat in its daily intake. The detailed results of this experiment were as follows (rest SBP):

- HV-MICT - reduction of 7.3 mm Hg
- HV-HIIT - reduction of 4.6 mm Hg
- LV-HIIT - reduction by 8.5 mm Hg

The research presented in the article by MartinezAguirre-Betolaza et al. (2020) adhered to the same methodology as the work reported in the publication by Gorostegi-Anduaga et al (2018).

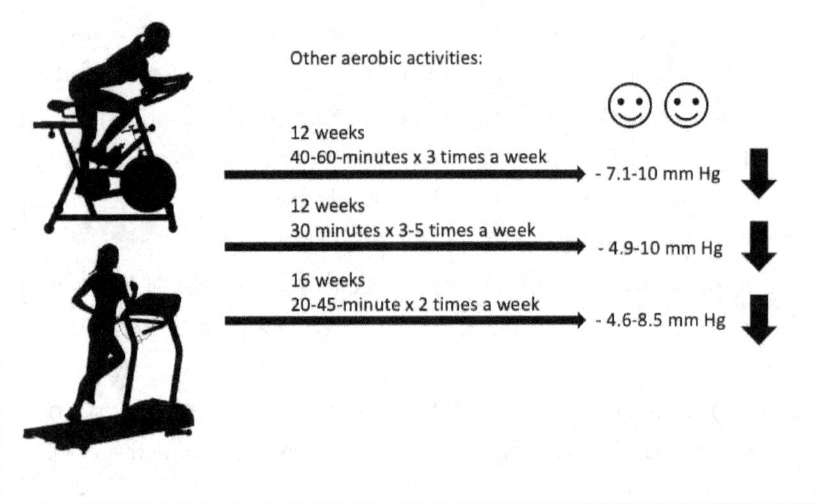

References

1. Barcellos, F. C., Del Vecchio, F. B., Reges, A., Mielke, G., Santos, I. S., Umpierre, D., ... & Hallal, P. C. (2018). Exercise in patients with hypertension and chronic kidney disease: a randomized controlled trial. Journal of human hypertension, 32(6), 397-407.

2. Gorostegi-Anduaga, I., Corres, P., MartinezAguirre-Betolaza, A., Pérez-Asenjo, J., Aispuru, G. R., Fryer, S. M., & Maldonado-Martin, S. (2018). Effects of different aerobic exercise programmes with nutritional intervention in sedentary adults with overweight/obesity and hypertension: EXERDIET-HTA study. European journal of preventive cardiology, 25(4), 343-353.

3. Lopes, S., Mesquita-Bastos, J., Garcia, C., Bertoquini, S., Ribau, V., Teixeira, M., ... & Ribeiro, F. (2021). Effect of exercise training on

ambulatory blood pressure among patients with resistant hypertension: a randomized clinical trial. JAMA cardiology, 6(11), 1317-1323.

4. MartinezAguirre-Betolaza, A., Mujika, I., Fryer, S. M., Corres, P., Gorostegi-Anduaga, I., Arratibel-Imaz, I., ... & Maldonado-Martin, S. (2020). Effects of different aerobic exercise programs on cardiac autonomic modulation and hemodynamics in hypertension: data from EXERDIET-HTA randomized trial. Journal of Human Hypertension, 34(10), 709-718.

5. Pagonas, N., Vlatsas, S., Bauer, F., Seibert, F. S., Zidek, W., Babel, N., ... & Westhoff, T. H. (2017). Aerobic versus isometric handgrip exercise in hypertension: a randomized controlled trial. Journal of hypertension, 35(11), 2199-2206.

2.2 ANAEROBIC TRAINING

In the following paragraphs, I will discuss the impact that anaerobic activity has on the lowering of hypertension levels. As this form of physical activity is not typically linked to the context of hypertension prevention, there are not a lot of publications on the subject, and the effects that can be achieved through anaerobic training are also not especially noteworthy. In my analysis, I took into consideration eight publications that investigated the impacts of various types of anaerobic physical activity, including the following:

- isometric training (3 studies),
- power training (1 study),
- resistance training (4 studies).

Only authors of publications describing resistance training obtained statistically significant effects on blood pressure, hence only this form of intervention is presented below.

2.2.1 Resistance training

The impact that resistance training has on blood pressure is described in the four publications that have been cited above. Two of the four very good results were obtained with a drop in mean blood pressure of 18 mm Hg (Pires et al., 2020) and 15 mm Hg (Taati et al. 2021). Statistically significant effects, although less than 7 mm Hg, were obtained by Heffernan et al. (2013) (6 mm Hg reduction) and Son et al. (2020) (3 mm Hg reduction).

Resistance training - how was the intervention conducted?

Single training sessions were applied by the authors of the study that was published by Pires et al. (2020), which was previously covered in the section on aerobic exercise. The resistance training program included 6 exercises, completed in 4 sets, with a total of 12 submaximal repetitions. The intensity of the workout was moderate (3-5 on the adapted Borg scale). These exercises were as follows:

- chair squat
- bench press on a vertical bench
- knee raise squat
- sit-up rowing
- dorsiflexion and sole flexion
- shoulder adduction.

There was a one-minute pause between each set and exercise. Muscle contractions, both concentric and eccentric, were carried out at a speed that was considered to be moderate, with each contraction taking around 2 seconds to complete. It was also stressed to the participants how important it was to avoid performing the Valsalva maneuver.

In the earlier section on the effects of green tea drinking on blood pressure, I partially discussed the approach that Taati et al. (2021) employed in their study. The authors of this study divided the hypertensive female volunteers, who ranged in age from 35 to 55 years old, into three groups: one group received only green tea, one group received both green tea and resistance training, and the last group only underwent resistance training. The duration of the intervention was 9 weeks. In the afternoon, twice a week, participants engaged in resistance training (4-6 p.m.). The training started out with a warm-up that consisted of walking and static stretching for ten minutes. The following exercises were then carried out by the participants: bench press, leg press, lat pulldown, knee extension, biceps curl, and leg curl. Participants completed two sets of ten repetitions at an intensity equal to fifty percent of their 1RM. The authors used the following formula to determine the RM (repetition maximum) for each subject: weight (kg)/[1.0278 - (0.0278 x number of repetitions)]. The time that passed between each set and circuit was exactly two minutes.

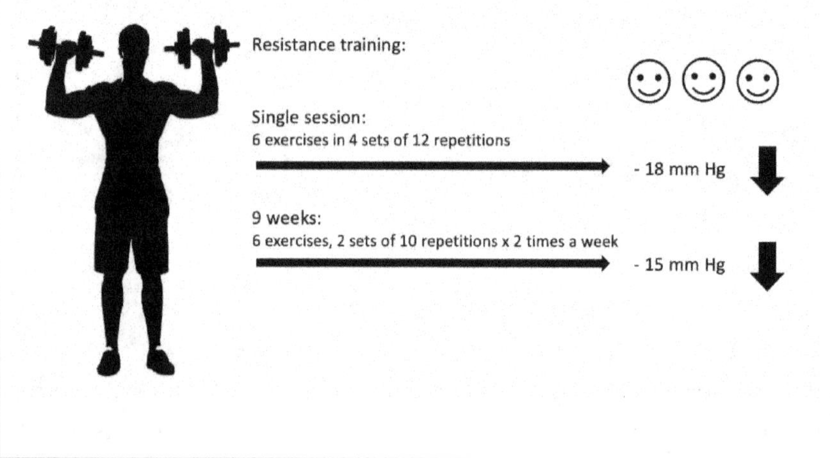

What you should know

- The power of baseball players was found to increase by an average of fifteen percent over the course of a season if the players ran eight wind sprints lasting between twenty and thirty seconds, three times per week (Rhea et al. 2008).

- Anaerobic activities, like aerobic exercises, have been found to have a beneficial effect on lipid metabolism and lipid profile (Patel et al. 2017).

- The findings provide support to the hypothesis that strength training can be just as beneficial as aerobic training in enhancing the physical abilities that contribute to functional mobility in later years. In addition, increased physical activity was associated with some mood enhancement (Martins et al. 2011).

- Your body's capacity to handle lactic acid can be improved through regular anaerobic training that takes you beyond your anaerobic threshold. This raises your lactic threshold, which is the point during which you begin to feel the effects of fatigue (Ghosh 2004).

- Training at a high intensity for short bursts may be beneficial for considerably improving both anaerobic and aerobic energy supply systems. This is likely achieved by imposing intense stimuli on both of these energy supply systems (Tabata et al. 1996).

- According to a review of research on the topic, anaerobic training at a high intensity on an intermittent basis provides a higher reduction in belly fat than continuous aerobic training does at equivalent levels of energy expenditure (Kuo and Harris 2016).

References

1. Ghosh, A. K. (2004). Anaerobic threshold: its concept and role in endurance sport. The Malaysian journal of medical sciences: MJMS, 11(1), 24.
2. Heffernan, K. S., Yoon, E. S., Sharman, J. E., Davies, J. E., Shih, Y. T., Chen, C. H., ... & Jae, S. Y. (2013). Resistance exercise training reduces arterial reservoir pressure in older adults with prehypertension and hypertension. Hypertension Research, 36(5), 422-427.
3. Kuo, C. H., & Harris, M. B. (2016). Abdominal fat reducing outcome of exercise training: fat burning or hydrocarbon source redistribution?. Canadian Journal of Physiology and Pharmacology, 94(7), 695-698.
4. Martins, R., Pindus, D., Cumming, S., Teixeira, A., & Veríssimo, M. (2011). Effects of strength and aerobic-based training on functional

fitness, mood and the relationship between fatness and mood in older adults. The Journal of sports medicine and physical fitness, 51(3), 489-496.

5. Patel, H., Alkhawam, H., Madanieh, R., Shah, N., Kosmas, C. E., & Vittorio, T. J. (2017). Aerobic vs anaerobic exercise training effects on the cardiovascular system. World journal of cardiology, 9(2), 134.

6. Pires, N. F., Coelho-Júnior, H. J., Gambassi, B. B., de Faria, A. P. C., Ritter, A. M. V., de Andrade Barboza, C., ... & Júnior, H. M. (2020). Combined aerobic and resistance exercises evokes longer reductions on ambulatory blood pressure in resistant hypertension: a randomized crossover trial. Cardiovascular therapeutics, 2020.

7. Rhea, M. R., Oliverson, J. R., Marshall, G., Peterson, M. D., Kenn, J. G., & Ayllón, F. N. (2008). Noncompatibility of power and endurance training among college baseball players. The Journal of Strength & Conditioning Research, 22(1), 230-234.

8. Son, W. M., Pekas, E. J., & Park, S. Y. (2020). Twelve weeks of resistance band exercise training improves age-associated hormonal decline, blood pressure, and body composition in postmenopausal women with stage 1 hypertension: a randomized clinical trial. Menopause, 27(2), 199-207.

9. Taati, B., Arazi, H., & Kheirkhah, J. (2021). Interaction effect of green tea consumption and resistance training on office and ambulatory cardiovascular parameters in women with high-normal/stage 1 hypertension. The Journal of Clinical Hypertension, 23(5), 978-986.

10. Tabata, I., Nishimura, K., Kouzaki, M., Hirai, Y., Ogita, F., Miyachi, M., & Yamamoto, K. (1996). Effects of moderate-intensity endurance and high-intensity intermittent training on anaerobic capacity and VO~ 2~ m~ a~ x. Medicine and science in sports and exercise, 28, 1327-1330.

2.3 COMBINED TRAINING

This part of the book describes various publications that, for the most part, discuss mixed physical activity, which is frequently a blend of aerobic and anaerobic activities. The following categories of interventions were included in the research that was carried out on 10 analyzed publications:

- qigong which is a set of exercises from ancient China (1 study),
- taekwondo (1 study),
- whole-body vibration exercise training (2 studies),
- others, including a combination of aerobic and strength training, one session of self-selected exercise (SSE)-intensity, a 12-week physical activity counselling intervention, and a combination of aerobic and resistance training (6 studies, in total).

2.3.1 Qigong

Xiao et al. (2016) conducted a study in which they invited Chinese subjects to participate. During the duration of the investigation, the participants were required to attend Ba duan jin Qigong Group lessons for a period of six months. The individuals' blood pressure decreased by an average of 20.2 mm Hg.

Qigong - how was the intervention conducted?

Participants attended classes 5 times a week for 6 months. Sessions included:

- 5-minute warm-up,
- 30 minutes of Qigong exercise,
- 5-minute cool-down.

There is a lack of specific information regarding this intervention within the published work, with the exception of broad guidelines from the Chinese Health Qigong Association.

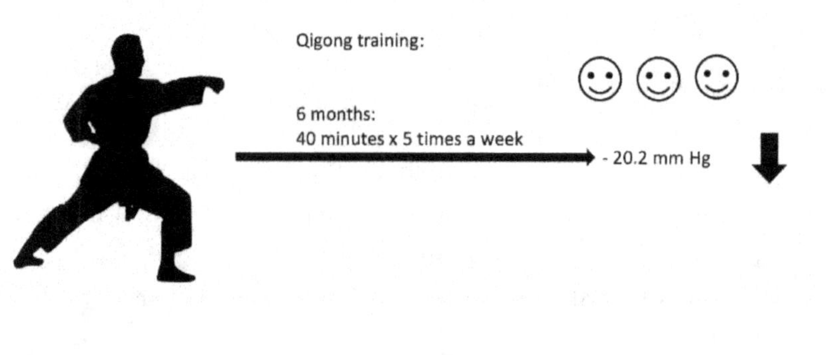

What you should know

- In studies where Qigong was compared to an inactive control, it was shown that depressive symptoms improved significantly (Tsang et al. 2006).
- The results of a one-month Qigong intervention showed significant improvements in a number of immune-related

blood markers, including the total number of leukocytes, the number of eosinphils, the number and percentage of monocytes, when compared to the results of treatment with the standard of care (Manzaneque et al. 2009).

- After participating in the trial for a period of four months, 64 individuals who suffered from chronic fatigue reported improvements in the severity of their symptoms. They had improved mental functioning and experienced less fatigue than individuals who did not undergo qigong training (Ho et al. 2012).

References

1. Ho, R. T., Chan, J. S., Wang, C. W., Lau, B. W., So, K. F., Yuen, L. P., ... & Chan, C. L. (2012). A randomized controlled trial of qigong exercise on fatigue symptoms, functioning, and telomerase activity in persons with chronic fatigue or chronic fatigue syndrome. Annals of Behavioral Medicine, 44(2), 160-170.
2. Manzaneque, J. M., Vera, F. M., Rodriguez, F. M., Garcia, G. J., Leyva, L., & Blanca, M. J. (2009). Serum cytokines, mood and sleep after a qigong program: is qigong an effective psychobiological tool?. Journal of Health Psychology, 14(1), 60-67.
3. Tsang, H. W., Fung, K. M., Chan, A. S., Lee, G., & Chan, F. (2006). Effect of a qigong exercise programme on elderly with depression. International Journal of Geriatric Psychiatry: A journal of the psychiatry of late life and allied sciences, 21(9), 890-897.
4. Xiao, C., Yang, Y., & Zhuang, Y. (2016). Effect of health Qigong Ba Duan Jin on blood pressure of individuals with essential hypertension. Journal of the American Geriatrics Society, 64(1), 211-213.

2.3.2 Taekwondo

Lee et al. (2019) described a 12-week taekwondo training program for postmenopausal women with hypertension stage 2. The average blood pressure of these participants decreased by 13 mm Hg.

Taekwondo - how was the intervention conducted?
Taekwondo training took place for an hour a day, three days a

week. During the first four weeks of training, the intensity of the exercise was kept at 30–40% of the participant's max HR, and then it was gradually increased up to 50–60% during the final four weeks of training. Before taking part in the experiment, each participant had previously engaged in taekwondo training at their schools. During the training, participants were required to wear protective gear for their bodies. The following are the components that made up the training:

- 10 minutes - dynamic stretching warm-up,
- 40 minutes - Taekwondo training:
    - kicks, punches, steps and step-sparring while facing an opponent (either an instructor or another participant),
    - remaining time - practicing Taekwondo forms and then walked, jogged or ran, depending on what intensity was desired,
- 10 minutes - static stretching cool-down.

Components of 40 minute Taekwondo training:
- Kicks: front kick, Round house kick, Side kick, Axe kick, Base kick, Turn-kick, Nara kick
- Punches: Reverse punch, Jab, Hook punch, Upper cut, Back fist, Hammer fist
- Steps: Forward-back step, One-two step
- Step Sparring: Tactical forward-back step, Tactical one-two step
- Taekwondo Forms: Palgwe, Taegeuk
- Aerobic Training: Walking, Jogging, Running

Taekwondo training program progression:
- 10 minutes - warm up - 1-12 weeks
- 40 minutes - Taekwondo Training Program:
    - 1-4 weeks, intensity: 30-40% max HR,

approximately 96-104 heart rate

- o 5-8 weeks, intensity: 40-50% max HR, approximately 105-112 heart rate
- o 9-12 weeks, intensity: 50-60% max HR, approximately 113-122 heart rate

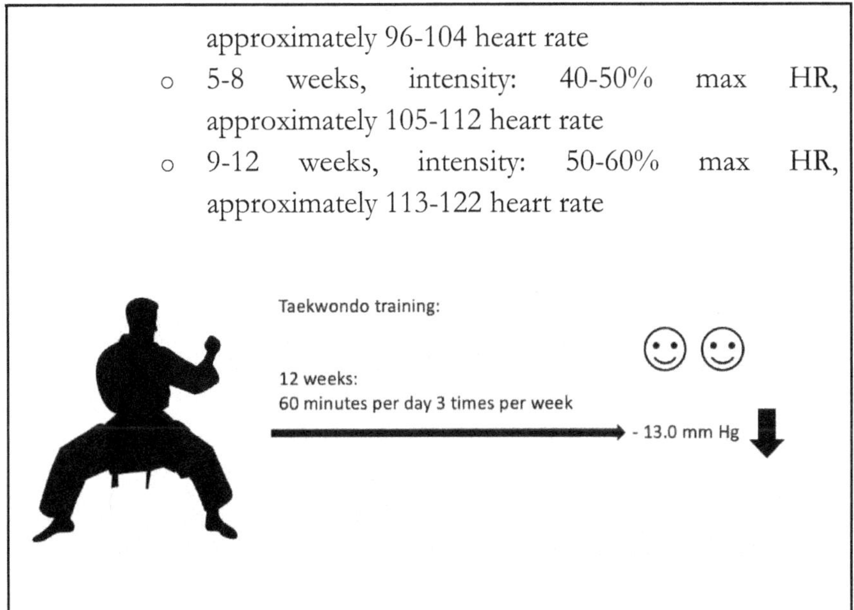

What you should know

- According to the findings, practicing a martial art is able to boost a person's strength in both the flexors and the extensors of the leg. In addition to this, their reaction times to acoustic stimuli are significantly quicker (Donovan et al. 2006).
- In a relatively short amount of time, low frequency taekwondo training in adolescent females promotes favorable changes in skeletal muscular fitness, flexibility, and body composition (Kim et al. 2011a).
- Participants who pursued Taekwondo as a serious form of recreation reported high levels of both life happiness and perceived health (Kim et al. 2011b).

References

1. Donovan, O. O., Cheung, J., Catley, M., McGregor, A. H., & Strutton, P. H. (2006). An investigation of leg and trunk strength and reaction times of hard-style martial arts practitioners. Journal of sports science & medicine, 5(CSSI), 5.

2. Kim, H. B., Stebbins, C. L., Chai, J. H., & Song, J. K. (2011a). Taekwondo training and fitness in female adolescents. Journal of sports sciences, 29(2), 133-138.

3. Kim, J., Dattilo, J., & Heo, J. (2011b). Taekwondo participation as serious leisure for life satisfaction and health. Journal of Leisure Research, 43(4), 545-559.

4. Lee, S. H., Scott, S. D., Pekas, E. J., Lee, S., Lee, S. H., & Park, S. Y. (2019). Taekwondo training reduces blood catecholamine levels and arterial stiffness in postmenopausal women with stage-2 hypertension: randomized clinical trial. Clinical and Experimental Hypertension, 41(7), 675-681.

2.3.3 Whole-body vibration exercise training

Exercise training with whole-body vibration was shown to reduce blood pressure in postmenopausal women in two trials that were carried out in the United States by Figueroa et al. (2014a, 2014b). Following an intervention that lasted for 6 and 12 weeks, a mean drop in blood pressure of 10 mm Hg and 12 mm Hg was found, respectively.

Whole-body vibration exercise training - how was the intervention conducted?

In the study that was carried out and described by Figueroa et al. (2014a), the participants were postmenopausal women who were around 56 years old and had a BMI (body mass index) of roughly 33.9. During the course of the study, participants took part in three supervised workout sessions per week, each of which was spaced out by a minimum of 48 hours. The training included standing leg exercises on a whole-body vibration platform. The exercises included both dynamic and static half squats and lunges at 120 degrees at the knees (treating 180 degrees as full knee extension), squats at 90 degrees at the knees, and calf raises. Dynamic exercises were performed with slow movements at a rate of 2 seconds for the concentric phase and 3 seconds for the eccentric phase. The vibration intensity was increased by increasing the frequency (25-35 Hz) and amplitude (1 mm). The duration was gradually increased from 30 to 45 seconds and the number of series (1-2), and the resting time was kept at 60 seconds.

An intervention that lasted for 12 weeks and was performed three times per week was described by Figueroa et al. (2014b). Each training session included four standing leg exercises that were performed on a whole body vibration platform. Both the frequency (25-40 Hz) and amplitude of the vibration were cranked up to create a more intense shaking (1 -2 mm). The duration was increased progressively from 30 seconds to 60 seconds, the number of series was increased from one to six, and the rest interval was decreased from sixty seconds to thirty seconds.

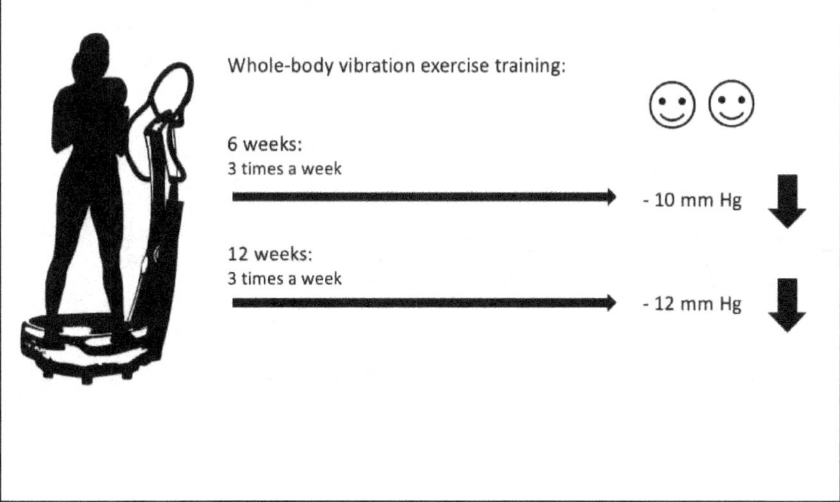

What you should know

- Whole-body vibration exercises have been shown to result in a number of positive outcomes. Increases in muscle strength and power, flexibility, and gait speed have been observed, along with increases in bone mineral density, balance, and quality of life, as well as a reduction in pain and the risk of falling (Bemben et al. 2018).

- Whole-body vibration exercises could be an important intervention due to their safety and effectiveness since they are vital for the management of unwanted clinical conditions that are caused by aging. Additionally, there is a connection between whole-body vibration activities and lower overall costs of medical care (Bemben et al. 2018).

References

1. Bemben, D., Stark, C., Taiar, R., & Bernardo-Filho, M. (2018). Relevance of whole-body vibration exercises on muscle strength/power and bone of elderly individuals. Dose-Response, 16(4), 1559325818813066.
2. Figueroa, A., Kalfon, R., Madzima, T. A., & Wong, A. (2014a). Effects of whole-body vibration exercise training on aortic wave reflection and muscle strength in postmenopausal women with prehypertension and hypertension. Journal of Human Hypertension, 28(2), 118-122.
3. Figueroa, A., Kalfon, R., Madzima, T. A., & Wong, A. (2014b). Whole-body vibration exercise training reduces arterial stiffness in postmenopausal women with prehypertension and hypertension. Menopause, 21(2), 131-136.

2.3.4 Others

In this section, I have included several publications that address combination training, which often consists of a mix of aerobic exercise and resistance training. Pires et al. (2020) described the best result, which was a drop in blood pressure of 14.3-19.5 mm Hg; however, this was just the result of one training session. After 12 weeks of resistance and aerobic exercise, the blood pressure of the participants dropped by an average of 13.5 mm Hg, as found in an experiment that was described by Son et al. (2017). The remaining four publications revealed a negligible effect of the intervention:

- Guirado et al. (2012) - reduction of 6 mm Hg following combined aerobic and strength training for 6 months
- Caminiti et al. (2021) - blood pressure reduction of 3.1-4.9 mm Hg following 12 week resistance and aerobic training

- Costa et al. (2019) - fall of 3.4 mm Hg, 1 session of self-selected exercise (SSE)-intensity training
- Pedralli et al. (2020) - decrease in blood pressure by an average of 3.2 mm Hg, following an 8 week resistant and aerobic training intervention

---

Others - how was the intervention conducted?

The only two publications in which the effect of the intervention was satisfactory, in the sense that it resulted in a drop greater than 7 mm Hg, are the ones that were discussed above.

Results obtained by Pires et al. (2020) were described not only in this section but also in others. Brazilian individuals with resistant hypertension (RH) and nonresistant hypertension (NON-RH) took part in a single morning exercise session that was comprised of the following steps:

- 25 minutes of an aerobic session performed at 50-60% max HR
- resistance session in the form of 2 sets of 12 submaximal repetitions at moderate intensity

Postmenopausal women with hypertension and aged around 75 were chosen as the subjects of the study by Son et al. (2017). They went to the gym three times a week for a total of twelve weeks to take part in the program, which consisted of a mix of aerobic and resistance training. The intensity of the training session was increased by 10% every four weeks, taking it from 40% to 70% of the heart's reserve capacity (HRR). Sessions were held three times a week for a total of 12 weeks, and each lasted approximately an hour and a half. The following were the components of each session:

- 5 minutes - warm-up consisted of static stretching,
- 20 minutes - various resistant band exercises:
    - upper: seated rows, biceps curl, shoulder flexion,

> elbow flexion, pushup,
>   - lower: hip flexion, hip extension, calf raise, leg press, squat,
> - 30 minutes of walking,
> - 5 minutes - cooldown consisted of static stretching.
>
> In weeks 1 to 4, exercise intensity increased from 40% to 50% HRR and from 60% to 70% in weeks 9 to 12.
>
> 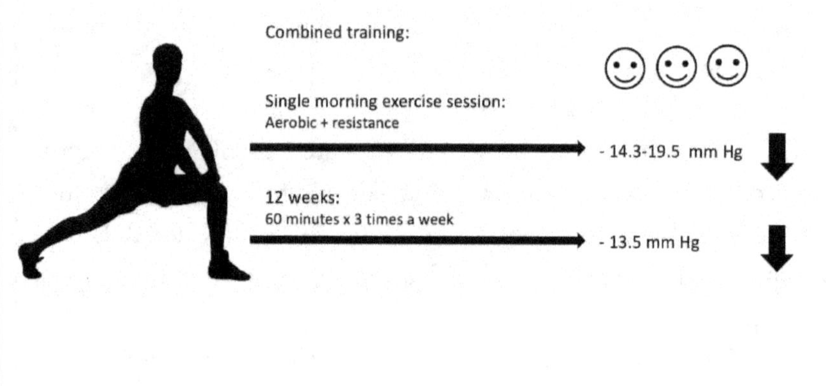
>

What you should know

- Studies have shown that combined training, which consists of aerobic and resistance exercising, results in greater improvements in total strength and fitness than any exercise modality conducted alone (Alberga et al. 2016, Santos et al. 2012).
- Twelve weeks of combination exercise increased adolescents' muscular and cardiorespiratory fitness and decreased their body fat percentage (Mendonça et al. 2022).

References

1. Alberga, A. S., Prud'homme, D., Sigal, R. J., Goldfield, G. S., Hadjiyannakis, S., Phillips, P., ... & Kenny, G. P. (2016). Effects of aerobic training, resistance training, or both on cardiorespiratory and musculoskeletal fitness in adolescents with obesity: the HEARTY trial. Applied Physiology, Nutrition, and Metabolism, 41(3), 255-265.

2. Caminiti, G., Iellamo, F., Mancuso, A., Cerrito, A., Montano, M., Manzi, V., & Volterrani, M. (2021). Effects of 12 weeks of aerobic versus combined aerobic plus resistance exercise training on short-term blood pressure variability in patients with hypertension. Journal of Applied Physiology, 130(4), 1085-1092.

3. Costa, I. B. B., Schwade, D., Macêdo, G. A. D., Browne, R. A. V., Farias-Junior, L. F., Freire, Y. A., ... & Costa, E. C. (2019). Acute antihypertensive effect of self-selected exercise intensity in older women with hypertension: a crossover trial. Clinical Interventions in Aging, 14, 1407.

4. Guirado, G. N., Damatto, R. L., Matsubara, B. B., Roscani, M. G., Fusco, D. R., Cicchetto, L. A., ... & Okoshi, M. P. (2012). Combined exercise training in asymptomatic elderly with controlled hypertension: effects on functional capacity and cardiac diastolic function. Medical science monitor: international medical journal of experimental and clinical research, 18(7), CR461.

5. Mendonça, F. R., de Faria, W. F., da Silva, J. M., Massuto, R. B., Dos Santos, G. C., Correa, R. C., ... & Neto, A. S. (2022). Effects of aerobic exercise combined with resistance training on health-related physical fitness in adolescents: A randomized controlled trial. Journal of Exercise Science & Fitness, 20(2), 182-189.

6. Pedralli, M. L., Marschner, R. A., Kollet, D. P., Neto, S. G., Eibel, B., Tanaka, H., & Lehnen, A. M. (2020). Different exercise training modalities produce similar endothelial function improvements in individuals with prehypertension or hypertension: A randomized clinical trial. Scientific reports, 10(1), 1-9.

7. Pires, N. F., Coelho-Júnior, H. J., Gambassi, B. B., de Faria, A. P. C., Ritter, A. M. V., de Andrade Barboza, C., ... & Júnior, H. M. (2020). Combined aerobic and resistance exercises evokes longer reductions on ambulatory blood pressure in resistant hypertension: a randomized crossover trial. Cardiovascular therapeutics, 2020.

8. Santos, A. P., Marinho, D. A., Costa, A. M., Izquierdo, M., & Marques, M. C. (2012). The effects of concurrent resistance and endurance training follow a detraining period in elementary school students. The Journal of Strength & Conditioning Research, 26(6), 1708-1716.

9. Son, W. M., Sung, K. D., Cho, J. M., & Park, S. Y. (2017). Combined exercise reduces arterial stiffness, blood pressure, and blood markers for cardiovascular risk in postmenopausal women with hypertension. Menopause, 24(3), 262-268.

2.4 Summary of physical activity interventions - what works

To conclude the chapter on physical activity, it should be stated that it has a significant effect on lowering blood pressure. Particularly, it is evident that aerobic activity (31 out of 32 studies reviewed obtained a statistically significant outcome) and combined training (all 10 studies show a statistically significant blood pressure reducing impact) were effective. Only four of the eight publications analyzed in the section on anaerobic activity demonstrated a statistically significant effect on lowering blood pressure, and they all involved resistance training, whereas interventions involving isometric training and power training did not demonstrate this effect.

The most noteworthy of the interventions that were described in the chapter on aerobic physical activity were aquatic exercises, particularly training sessions in a heated pool, which, after a few weeks, had the effect of lowering blood pressure by an average of almost 20 mm Hg. Interval training, cycling, and Tai Chi also produced favorable outcomes. In addition, a single session of running on a treadmill dropped a person's blood pressure by 15.4 to 18 mm Hg, although prolonged interventions did not show such stunning results.

Resistance training, which is discussed in the section on anaerobic activity, was found to produce very good results in two studies, reducing blood pressure by an average of 18 mm Hg (although this was only the effect of a single session) and by 15 mm Hg. In the other two interventions, the outcomes were far less impressive.

In the chapter on combined training, the best outcome was achieved with a six-month intervention that comprised Qigong group lessons. The average reduction in blood pressure was greater than 20 mm Hg, which was the best outcome for physical activity throughout the period under consideration. Taekwondo and the combination of aerobic activity and resistance training, which is discussed in the section titled "Others," both had noteworthy benefits.

Figure 6 illustrates the highest values of blood pressure reduction that can be achieved by each of the several types of interventions. This chart does not show the full picture, but it does provide you with a general understanding of the different types of physical activity that have a strong possibility of lowering hypertension.

The same list of interventions is displayed in Figure 7; however, the plots in this figure only include the three primary categories of physical activity: aerobic, anaerobic, and combined. There are four examples of combination training in the top 10, compared to five examples of aerobic training and just one example of anaerobic training. This again demonstrates the prevalence of combined and aerobic activity over anaerobic training. There were three times less papers on combined training than there were on aerobic training; however, there are almost as many interventions from both types of activity in the top 10. This is something that should be mentioned.

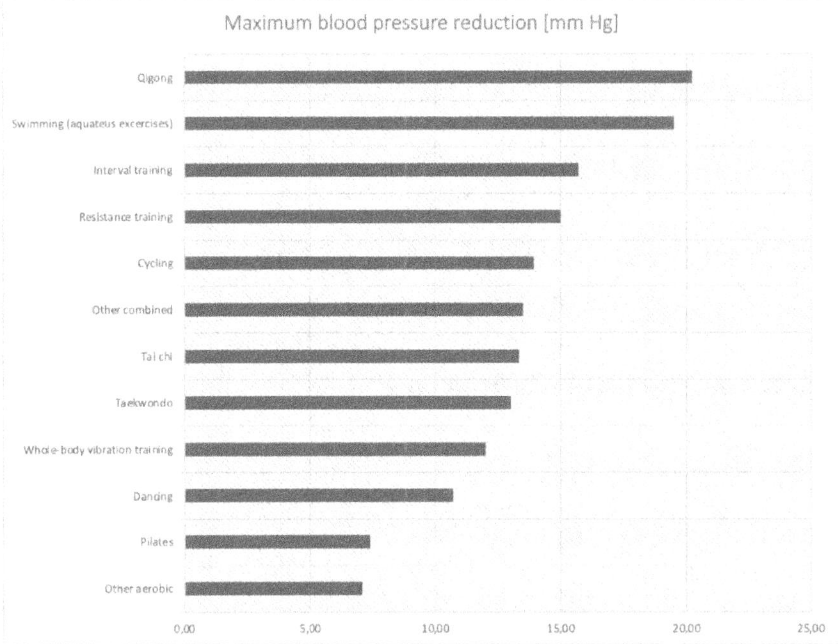

Figure 6. The highest values of blood pressure reduction achieved by selected interventions in the area of physical activity. Despite the fact that those interventions were also discussed in the text, the plot does not include the data from any of the training sessions in which they were conducted as single training sessions.

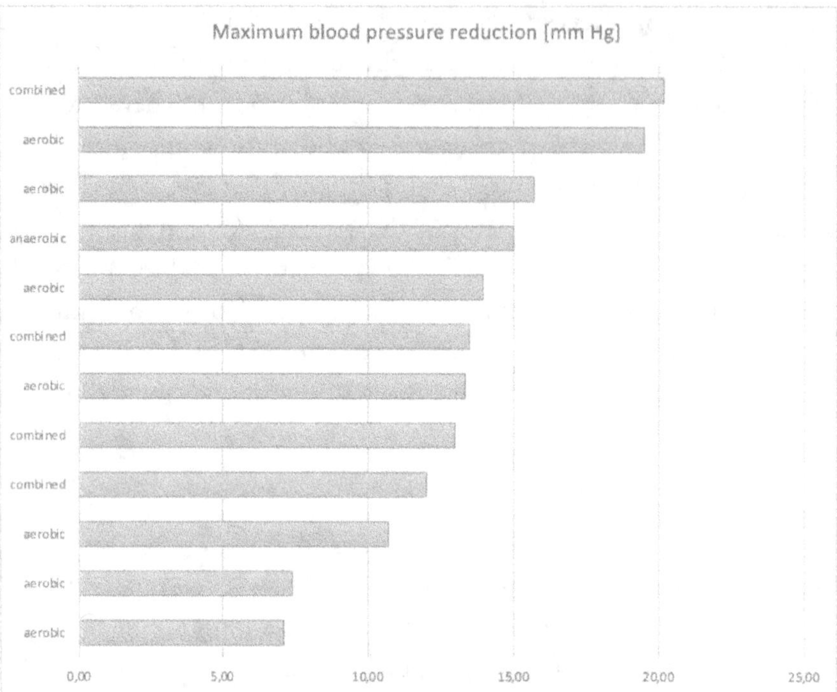

Figure 7. The highest values of blood pressure reduction shown in the context of the type of physical activity that describes the intervention. The position on the plot corresponds exactly to the interventions placed on the earlier plot.

PART 3. OTHER INTERVENTIONS

This section is the fourth part of this book, describing experiments that measured the effects of specific interventions on blood pressure. I have included all of the interventions that cannot be categorized in any of the other sections in this part. The effects of the following factors are described below:

- acupressure (2 studies),
- acupuncture (5 studies),
- behavioral or lifestyle modifications (9 studies),
- breathing training (9 studies),
- marital status (1 study),
- sauna (1 study),
- social media education (1 study),
- stress management (2 studies),
- yoga (7 studies).

Only social media education had no significant effect on participants' blood pressure among the factors described. Within each type of intervention that was examined, at least one publication out of those that were explored suggested that there was an effect on the subject's blood pressure.

3.1 Acupressure

Two studies, one by Bicer et al. (2021) and one by Yeh et al. (2015), were conducted to investigate the impact that acupressure has on blood pressure. In the first study, participants who underwent auricular acupressure for a period of ten weeks did not see a drop in their blood pressure. In contrast, Yeh et al. (2015) discovered that after four weeks of acupressure treatment in Turkish individuals with essential hypertension, there was a significant reduction in blood pressure of an average of -11.44 mm Hg.

Acupressure - how was the intervention conducted?

The intervention, which lasted for four weeks, involved applying acupressure with an electrostimulation device to the Neiguan (P6) acupuncture point on the wrist. This point is located approximately two fingers away from the inner curve of the wrist, on the line of the middle finger, and in the space between the tendons of the palmaris longus and the flexor carpi radialis (Yeh et al. 2015). At regular intervals of 5 seconds and at a frequency of 10 Hz, the device delivered pressure to the point of interest. The sessions continued for one month, during which time they were carried out seven days a week for a duration of half an hour each.

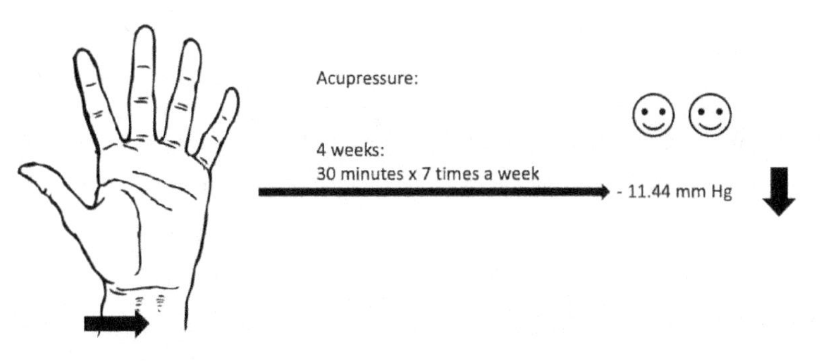

What you should know

- Some medical studies have suggested that acupressure can help with symptoms like nausea and vomiting, sleeplessness, low back pain, migraines, and constipation. However, it is still officially recognized as not being fully proven (Lee and Frazier 2011).

- According to the findings of the study, auricular acupressure could be beneficial for weight loss. However, these findings also need to be confirmed by additional detailed research (Huang et al. 2019).

References

1. Biçer, S., Ünsal, A., Tasci, S., Demir, G., & Ceyhan, Y. S. (2021). The effect of acupressure on blood pressure level and pulse rate in individuals with essential hypertension: a randomized controlled trial. Holistic Nursing Practice, 35(1), 40-48.
2. Huang, C. F., Guo, S. E., & Chou, F. H. (2019). Auricular acupressure for overweight and obese individuals: a systematic review and meta-analysis. Medicine, 98(26).
3. Lee, E. J., & Frazier, S. K. (2011). The efficacy of acupressure for symptom management: a systematic review. Journal of pain and symptom management, 42(4), 589-603.
4. Yeh, M. L., Chang, Y. C., Huang, Y. Y., & Lee, T. Y. (2015). A randomized controlled trial of auricular acupressure in heart rate variability and quality of life for hypertension. Complementary Therapies in Medicine, 23(2), 200-209.

3.2 Acupuncture

Acupuncture is regarded as a centuries-old way of treating numerous disorders by inserting specific needles into the patient's body. Five publications (Huang et al. 2022, Liu et al. 2015, Silva et al. 2020, Zhang et al. 2021, Zheng et al. 2019) investigated the effects of acupuncture on blood pressure. Of these publications, one found no statistically significant effects, three found effects that were not very large (a reduction in blood pressure by an average of 4.8-6.3 mm Hg), and only one found effects above 7 mm Hg (8.6 mm Hg).

Acupuncture - how was the intervention conducted?

South Korean participants with prehypertension and stage I hypertension were involved in the study by Liu et al. (2015). The study was conducted on subjects who were residents of South Korea. The patient received acupuncture on a twice-weekly basis for a total of eight weeks, after which there was a follow-up period of four weeks during which no treatment was administered. Stainless steel needles with a diameter of 0.20 mm and a length of 30 mm were used during the intervention. In addition, as mentioned by the study authors, "participants were given de qi sensation via manipulation right after inserting needle into the skin, plus 20 min of needle-retaining time." All treatments were performed by experts who selected acupuncture points as bilateral ST36, PC6, LR3, SP4, LI11. It is worth noting here that after 8 weeks of intervention the blood pressure was not significantly different, only after another 4 weeks (a total of 12 weeks from the start of the intervention) blood pressure was significantly lower by an average of 8.6 mm Hg.

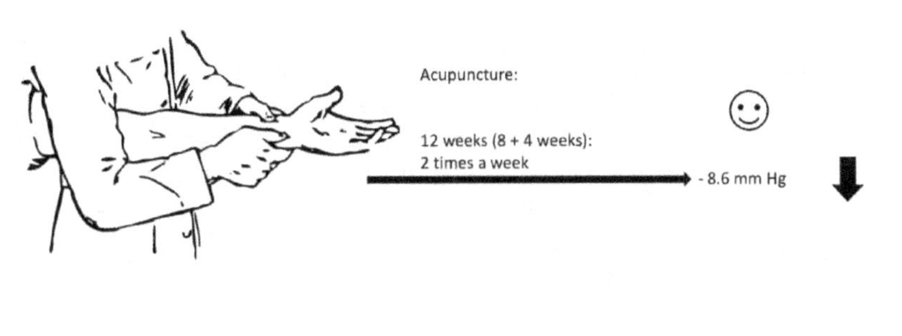

What you should know

- Acupuncture has been the subject of a significant amount of research, particularly for the treatment of pain associated with osteoarthritis and knee discomfort, as well as headaches. However, researchers are just starting to understand whether or not acupuncture can help relieve a variety of health problems. When conducted by a competent, well-trained practitioner using sterile needles, acupuncture is usually considered to be safe. Acupuncture that is not conducted correctly can result in major adverse consequences. (National Center for Complementary and Integrative Health, 2016).

- According to the findings of several studies, a great number of acupuncture points are located at places where stimulation can influence the activity of a number of different sensory neurons. These locations are also referred to as receptive fields. It is possible that the physical stimulation caused by the insertion of the needle at certain areas will influence the way that the central nervous system and muscles process pain, as well as increase the flow of blood to certain sections of the body (Quiroz-González et al. 2017).

References

1. Huang, K. Y., Chang, C. H., Yu, K. C., & Hsu, C. H. (2022). Assessment of quality of life and activities of daily living among elderly patients with hypertension and impaired physical mobility in home health care by antihypertensive drugs plus acupuncture: A CONSORT-compliant, randomized controlled trial. Medicine, 101(11), e29077.
2. Liu, Y., Park, J. E., Shin, K. M., Lee, M., Jung, H. J., Kim, A. R., ... & Choi, S. M. (2015). Acupuncture lowers blood pressure in mild hypertension patients: a randomized, controlled, assessor-blinded pilot trial. Complementary Therapies in Medicine, 23(5), 658-665.
3. National Center for Complementary and Integrative Health. Acupuncture: In Depth. (n.d.). NCCIH. Retrieved September 8, 2022, from https://www.nccih.nih.gov/health/acupuncture-in-depth
4. Silva, M. V. F., Lustosa, T. C., Arai, V. J., Couto Patriota, T. L., Lira, M. P., Lins-Filho, O. L., ... & Pedrosa, R. P. (2020). Effects of acupuncture on obstructive sleep apnea severity, blood pressure control and quality of life in patients with hypertension: A randomized controlled trial. Journal of sleep research, 29(2), e12954.
5. Quiroz-González, S., Torres-Castillo, S., López-Gómez, R. E., & Estrada, I. J. (2017). Acupuncture points and their relationship with multireceptive fields of neurons. Journal of Acupuncture and Meridian Studies, 10(2), 81-89.
6. Zhang, J., Lyu, T., Yang, Y., Wang, Y., Zheng, Y., Qu, S., ... & Huang, Y. (2021). Acupuncture at LR3 and KI3 shows a control effect on essential hypertension and targeted action on cerebral regions related to blood

pressure regulation: a resting state functional magnetic resonance imaging study. Acupuncture in Medicine, 39(1), 53-63.

7. Zheng, H., Li, J., Li, Y., Zhao, L., Wu, X., Chen, J., ... & Liang, F. R. (2019). Acupuncture for patients with mild hypertension: a randomized controlled trial. The Journal of Clinical Hypertension, 21(3), 412-420.

3.3 Behavioral or lifestyle modification

Nine publications described interventions that their authors explained as behavioral or lifestyle modification training (Blumenthal et al. 2021, Friedberg et al. 2015, Liang et al. 2015, Ma et al. 2014, Ma et al. 2021, Nolan et al. 2012, Shamsi et al. 2021, Vamvakis et al. 2020, and Zou et al. 2017). Some of these interventions took the form of regular training sessions, whereas others took the form of simple educational programs. It's interesting to note that these interventions were often much longer than the ones in the other sections; the shortest one lasted for two months. Only one of the studies, which lasted for a total of eight weeks and consisted of behavioral training as the intervention, failed to demonstrate a statistically significant reduction in blood pressure. In the other articles, a four-month intervention that included a lifestyle intervention in the form of a continuous care model was successful in lowering the participants' blood pressure by up to 15.2 mm Hg. The methodology of the studies in which the effect of lowering blood pressure was more than 7 mm Hg on average is discussed below, and this applies to five of the nine publications that are evaluated in this area.

Behavioral or lifestyle modification - how was the intervention conducted?

The authors of the study that was published by Shamsi et al. (2021) (which resulted in a 15.2 mm Hg reduction in blood pressure) had the objective of lowering the amount of sodium consumed through diet as well as blood pressure in hypertensive patients. They intended to accomplish this objective through the implementation of lifestyle changes. The Iranian volunteers, who ranged in age from 40 to 70 years, took part in an intervention that took place over a period of four months and consisted of the following stages:

- 1 session that lasted from around 20 to 40 minutes, included the following: familiarization of the patient and the nurse, explanation of the stages of the model, generation of motivation, explanation of the goals and how to implement the intervention, as well as the time and place of subsequent meetings.
- 8 sessions of 60 minutes each, twice a week - these were educational courses on hypertension and healthy lifestyles:
  - 3 sessions on hypertension, its effects, and the variables that put people at risk for cardiovascular disease.
  - 3 sessions on healthy eating with an emphasis on necessary dietary changes - the aim of these courses was to increase the intake of fruits and vegetables, nuts, whole grains products and legumes, encourage a diet rich in mono- and polyunsaturated fats, lean protein and low- and non-fat dairy; and reducing the overall intake of calories, desserts, processed foods, sugary beverages, saturated fats, and sodium chloride (<5 g/day) or sodium (<2 g/day).
  - 2 sessions on physical activity - the goal was to promote physical activity among participants and their families, including moderate-intensity aerobic exercise (usually for 20-30 minutes), such as walking and Pilates exercises.
- 12 consultation sessions of 40 minutes each, which were conducted once a week - participants were encouraged to continue a healthy lifestyle and adherence to treatment, patients were also monitored for acquired knowledge.

- At the end of the study, the effects of the intervention were evaluated by measuring the participants' blood pressure and determining how much salt they took in.

Vamvakis et al. (2020) designed a protocol in which participants received rigorous lifestyle treatment (diet plus exercise with monthly visits). Patients from Greece who were in an untreated stage I of hypertension were included in the study. In accordance with the guidelines provided by the European Society of Hypertension (ESH), the participants in the study were given information regarding diet (during a one-hour individual nutrition education session) and exercise. This information included the necessity of lowering salt consumption, the requirement of increasing physical activity, and the advantages of losing weight during the course of the 6-month study. In addition, each participant received an individualized diet plan to follow during the study (but details of the diet plan are missing). During the course of the experiment, there were monthly repeats of the in-depth sessions that lasted one hour each. Blood pressure dropped by an average of 11-14.6 mm Hg as a result of this intervention, however the exact range varied depending on how it was monitored (ambulatory, daytime, or office blood pressure).

Filipino Americans who lived in the Greater Philadelphia Area were the participants in the study that was detailed by Ma et al. (2021). The intervention consisted of holding two instructional sessions and then monitoring the outcomes of those sessions over a period of three months to determine their effectiveness. This intervention program was planned in close coordination with leaders of the Filipino-American community, who also took part in arranging the workshops. The educational sessions included the following topics:

- Center for Disease Control and Prevention (CDC) guidelines on physical activity and its benefits,

- statistics on physical activity participation in the US and among Filipinos,
- statistics on rates of high blood pressure among Filipinos,
- physical inactivity as a risk factor for chronic diseases,
- types of physical activity,
- physical activity and lowering blood pressure,
- use of a mobile app to track physical activity,
- barriers and strategies to engaging in physical activity,
- dietary sodium, sodium as a risk factor for hypertension, sodium intake guidelines.

During the workshop, attendees also learned how to make recipes for low-salt meals and had hands-on experience with a mobile app that monitors salt consumption. In addition, there were sessions of physical activity that lasted for a total of one hour and were led by an instructor who had the appropriate credentials. Participants were also given instructional materials on the importance of being physically active. The first session was a Zumba class, while the second session was yoga. After three months of this intervention, a decrease in blood pressure of 12.6 mm Hg was observed to have occurred.

In patients who had resistant hypertension, Blumenthal et al. (2021) wanted to determine whether or not a lifestyle intervention would have an influence on their blood pressure. Dietary counseling, behavioral weight management, and exercise were all components of the four-month program that the participants were required to take part in. In this study, one group was contrasted with another that had just undergone a single therapy session. The DASH diet, which included calorie and sodium restriction (less than 2300 mg per day), was presented to the participants. Each group counseling session lasted for half an hour and was held once a week under the direction of a clinical psychologist. The sessions focused on healthy eating patterns. During these sessions, motivational interviewing strategies were used in the form of reinforcing participants' motivation to choose appropriate products and overcome obstacles to following the DASH diet. These strategies were used in conjunction with a reinforcement of participants' motivation to choose appropriate products.

In addition, participants exercised three times per week for a duration ranging from 30 to 45 minutes at a heart rate that was between 70% and 85% of their initial heart rate reserve. These sessions were comprised of the following:

- 10 minutes of warm up exercises,
- 30-45 minutes of biking and/or walking (and eventually jogging),
- 10 minutes of cool down exercises.

Once a week, either just before or directly after one of the weekly exercise sessions, participants attended a session that focused on weight management strategies. Exercises for monitoring one's own hunger cues were a part of these sessions. Patients participated in these activities in order to learn how to make decisions while managing their hunger and fullness to the greatest extent possible. In the beginning, the participants were requied to meticulously record the quantity and type of food that they consumed, as well as their feelings of hunger before eating and fullness after eating. Later on, the number of days of monitoring was cut down, and they transitioned from using written appetite monitoring to mental monitoring (visualization). Participants' blood pressure decreased by an average of 12.5 mm Hg (clinic systolic BP) and by 7 mm Hg (24-hour ambulatory systolic BP).

The intervention, which was proposed by Ma et al. (2014) and took the form of counseling in the context of motivational interviewing, worked on changing patients' behaviors over the course of a period of six months. These behaviors included taking medications on time, maintaining healthy eating habits, engaging in regular physical activity, refraining from drinking and smoking, and managing stress. The following were some of the things that were included in the program:

- building relationships with patients,
- assessing and building motivation for behavior change,
- helping patients become aware of and address underlying ambivalence that blocks their behavior to change,
- searching for discrepancies between their values and current behaviors,
- building strategies for adherence to behavior change,
- analyzing the pros and cons of proposed behavioral changes,
- setting realistic and specific goals.

On the basis of the participants' consistent recording in their diaries, the nurses and the participants worked together to establish a set of goals that addressed a variety of aspects of the participant's physical and mental well-being, including their dietary routines, the medications they took, their level of physical activity, whether or not they drank alcohol or smoked. The sessions typically lasted between thirty and forty minutes and were repeated eight times spread out over a period of six months. The average blood pressure of the participants dropped by 7.81 mm Hg.

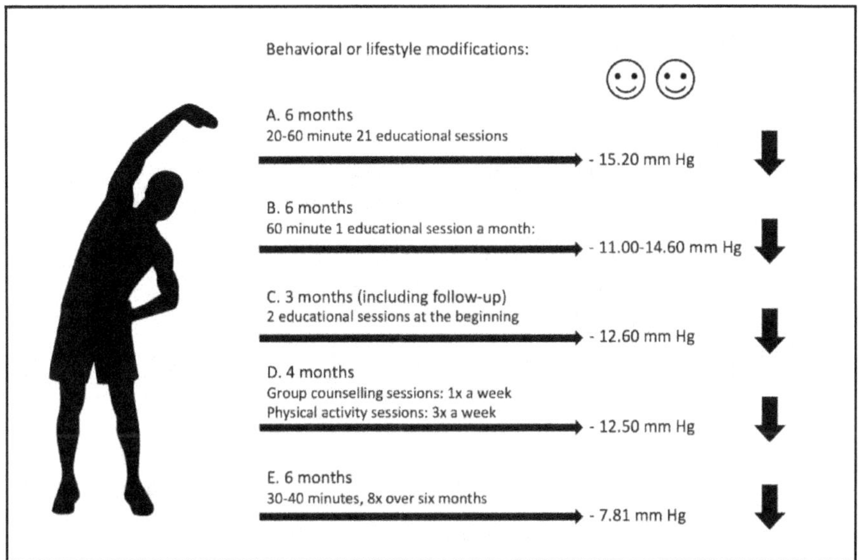

References

1. Blumenthal, J. A., Hinderliter, A. L., Smith, P. J., Mabe, S., Watkins, L. L., Craighead, L., ... & Sherwood, A. (2021). Effects of lifestyle modification on patients with resistant hypertension: results of the TRIUMPH randomized clinical trial. Circulation, 144(15), 1212-1226.

2. Friedberg, J. P., Rodriguez, M. A., Watsula, M. E., Lin, I., Wylie-Rosett, J., Allegrante, J. P., ... & Natarajan, S. (2015). Effectiveness of a tailored behavioral intervention to improve hypertension control: primary outcomes of a randomized controlled trial. Hypertension, 65(2), 440-446.

3. Liang, Y., Ehler, B. R., Hollenbeak, C. S., & Turner, B. J. (2015). Behavioral support intervention for uncontrolled hypertension: a complier average causal effect (CACE) analysis. Medical care, 53(2), e9-e15.

4. Ma, C., Zhou, Y., Zhou, W., & Huang, C. (2014). Evaluation of the effect of motivational interviewing counselling on hypertension care. Patient education and counseling, 95(2), 231-237.

5. Ma, G. X., Bhimla, A., Zhu, L., Beeber, M., Aczon, F., Tan, Y., ... & Gadegbeku, C. A. (2021). Development of an intervention to promote physical activity and reduce dietary sodium intake for preventing hypertension and chronic disease in Filipino Americans. Journal of racial and ethnic health disparities, 8(2), 283-292.

6. Nolan, R. P., Floras, J. S., Ahmed, L., Harvey, P. J., Hiscock, N., Hendrickx, H., & Talbot, D. (2012). Behavioural modification of the cholinergic anti-inflammatory response to C-reactive protein in patients with hypertension. Journal of Internal Medicine, 272(2), 161-169.

7. Shamsi, S. A., Salehzadeh, M., Ghavami, H., Asl, R. G., & Vatani, K. K. (2021). Impact of lifestyle interventions on reducing dietary sodium intake

and blood pressure in patients with hypertension: a randomized controlled trial. Turk Kardiyol Dern Ars, 49(2), 143-150.

8. Vamvakis, A., Gkaliagkousi, E., Lazaridis, A., Grammatikopoulou, M. G., Triantafyllou, A., Nikolaidou, B., ... & Douma, S. (2020). Impact of intensive lifestyle treatment (Diet plus exercise) on endothelial and vascular function, arterial stiffness and blood pressure in stage 1 hypertension: Results of the HINTreat randomized controlled trial. Nutrients, 12(5), 1326.

9. Zou, P., Dennis, C. L., Lee, R., & Parry, M. (2017). Dietary approach to stop hypertension with sodium reduction for Chinese Canadians (Dashna-CC): a pilot randomized controlled trial. The journal of nutrition, health & aging, 21(10), 1225-1232.

3.4 Breathing training

In the past decade, nine scientific articles have examined the relationship between breathing exercises and a reduction in blood pressure (Ghati et al. 2021, Hering et al. 2013, Landman et al. 2013, Sangthong et al. 2016, Telles et al. 2013, Thanalakshmi et al. 2020, Ubolsakka-Jones et al. 2017, 2018, 2019). No significant effect on blood pressure was found in two of the experiments, the effect on blood pressure in one of the experiments was small (Telles et al. 2013, reduction by 2.17-4.37 mm Hg), while the effect on blood pressure in other publications was either very good (reduction up to 17-18 mm Hg: Ubolsakka-Jones 2018, 2019, Sangthong et al. 2016, and Hering et al. 2013) or satisfactory (a reduction of more than 10 mm Hg was found.

Breathing training - how was the intervention conducted?
The study that was published by Hering et al. (2013) describes an intervention that took the form of a device-guided breathing training (device: RESPeRATE, Intercure Ltd.). This training lasted for a total of 8 weeks and led to a reduction in blood pressure that was approximately 18 mm Hg lower on average (office blood pressure). Interestingly, however, other pressure measurements did not indicate its reduction through this intervention. Men with newly

---

diagnosed hypertension participated in this study. In this study, participants were males who had recently been diagnosed with hypertension. A training session for device-guided breathing aimed to achieve 10 breaths per minute while accumulating 40 minutes of therapeutic breathing each week. The participants attended the sessions on a daily basis for a total of fifteen minutes.

Individuals who suffer from a condition known as "isolated systolic hypertension" were the subjects of a study that was conducted by Sangthong et al. (2016). The researchers intended to examine the effects of slow breathing training, both with and without an inspiratory load. Sessions were conducted once a day, every day, for a total of eight weeks at home. Participants from Thailand who agreed to take part in the study were separated into two groups for the intervention:

- loaded breathing - six breaths per minute, 18 cm H2O,
- unloaded breathing - six breaths per minute, no load.

The loaded group saw an average decrease in blood pressure of 18 mm Hg, while the unloaded group saw an average decrease in blood pressure of 11 mm Hg. The intervention required the participants to take lengthy breaths at a pace of six per minute while utilizing a pressure threshold incentive spirometer. The inspiratory resistance was calculated by measuring the amount of water that was contained within the bottle (load group: 18 cm H2O, no load group: there was no water in the device). The objective was to take a 4-second breath in and a 6-second breath out. The purpose of the training was to make use of the metronome initially; but, as participants gained experience and became more proficient, the metronome became less necessary, and eventually they were able to count in their heads. A single training session lasted for half an hour.

An analogous study was conducted by Ublosakka-Jones et al.

(2019), in which individuals with isolated systolic hypertension also undertook an 8-week intervention in the form of slow loaded breathing (25% maximal inspiratory pressure, 6 breaths per minute, 60 breaths every day) or deep breathing control. The first group used BreatheMAX inspiratory training apparatus to conduct their sessions, during which they subjected themselves to a load equal to 25% of their maximum inspiratory pressure. The challenge for the participants was to keep their breathing at a rate of six breaths per minute, with each inhale lasting four seconds and each exhale lasting six seconds. In this particular apparatus, the inspiratory resistance was determined by the amount of water that was contained within the container. The group that did the sessions with the device showed an average decrease in blood pressure of as much as 22 mm Hg, but there was also a decrease in blood pressure in the group that did deep breathing (control), so the result for the first group was 17 mm Hg after taking the result for the control group into account.

In the earlier experiment that was detailed by Ublosakka-Jones et al. (2018), the exact same methodology that was used in the aforementioned study was applied. The experiment produced very comparable outcomes, with participants' blood pressure dropping by 17 mm Hg on average (reduction by 20 mm Hg in the load group and by 3 mm Hg in a control deep breathing group).

Patients suffering from hypertension in India were given Sheetali pranayama breathing training as part of a specific kind of intervention that was detailed by Thanalakshmi et al. (2020). Patients were instructed to close their eyes and take deep breaths via their tongues, which were folded into the shape of a tube. Following that, they were required to exhale slowly, while doing so via both nostrils. After completing 10 of these breaths, participants were required to take a break for two minutes. The cycle of ten breaths followed by one rest should be completed no less than twenty times, and the total practice should take no less than half an hour each day. The training started at seven in the morning and continued until nine in the morning. As a consequence of this intervention, the participants' blood pressure dropped by a mean of 13.38 mm Hg.

The intervention that was described by Ublosakka-Jones et al. (2017), which featured slow breathing against an inspiratory resistance of 18 cm H2O, lasted for a total of 8 weeks, and had the effect of lowering blood pressure by an average of 10.6 mm Hg. Participants were instructed to inhale for a period of four seconds and exhale for a period of six seconds. The total duration of the session for the day was thirty minutes, and participants were to attend this session on a daily basis for the aforementioned period of eight weeks. It is important to note that the authors conducted their research on the same patients as Sangthong et al. did in their study (2016).

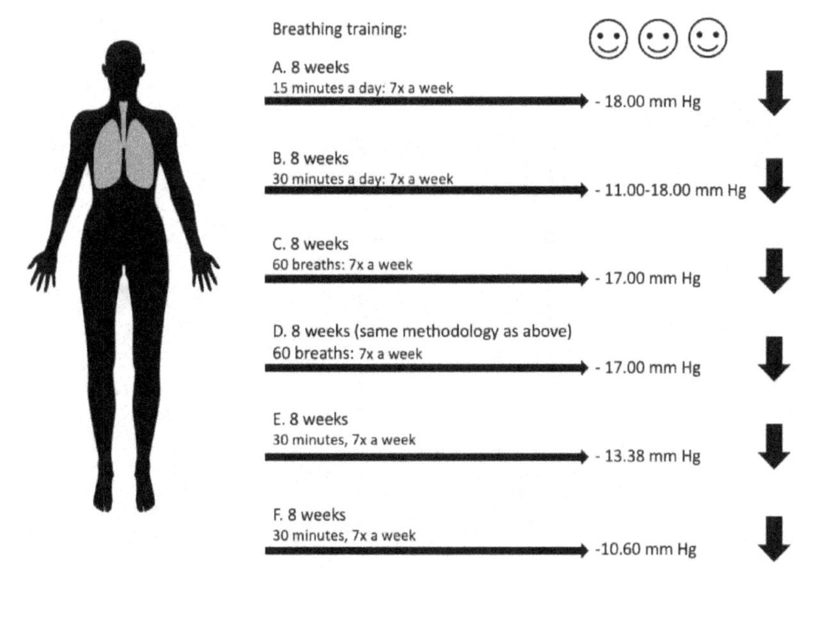

What you should know

- In elderly people, regular breathing exercises may be especially helpful in lowering their chance of developing cardiovascular disease (Craighead et al. 2021).

- Regular practice of breathing exercises has been linked to greater concentration and focus, as well as enhanced memory and improved decision-making ability (Sharma et al. 2014).

- Patients suffering from chronic lung disorders such as asthma, emphysema, bronchitis, and others have found that breathing exercises are of great benefit to their condition (Ubolnuar et al. 2019).

References

1. Craighead, D. H., Heinbockel, T. C., Freeberg, K. A., Rossman, M. J., Jackman, R. A., Jankowski, L. R., ... & Seals, D. R. (2021). Time-Efficient Inspiratory Muscle Strength Training Lowers Blood Pressure and Improves Endothelial Function, NO Bioavailability, and Oxidative Stress in Midlife/Older Adults With Above-Normal Blood Pressure. Journal of the American Heart Association, 10(13), e020980.

2. Ghati, N., Killa, A. K., Sharma, G., Karunakaran, B., Agarwal, A., Mohanty, S., ... & Pandey, R. M. (2021). A randomized trial of the immediate effect of bee-humming breathing exercise on blood pressure and heart rate variability in patients with essential hypertension. EXPLORE, 17(4), 312-319.

3. Hering, D., Kucharska, W., Kara, T., Somers, V. K., Parati, G., & Narkiewicz, K. (2013). Effects of acute and long-term slow breathing exercise on muscle sympathetic nerve activity in untreated male patients with hypertension. Journal of hypertension, 31(4), 739-746.

4. Landman, G. W., Drion, I., van Hateren, K. J., van Dijk, P. R., Logtenberg, S. J., Lambert, J., ... & Kleefstra, N. (2013). Device-guided breathing as treatment for hypertension in type 2 diabetes mellitus: a randomized, double-blind, sham-controlled trial. JAMA internal medicine, 173(14), 1346-1350.

5. Sangthong, B., Ubolsakka-Jones, C., Pachirat, O., & Jones, D. A. (2016). Breathing Training for Older Patients with Controlled Isolated Systolic Hypertension. Medicine and Science in Sports and Exercise, 48(9), 1641-1647.

6. Sharma, V. K., Rajajeyakumar, M., Velkumary, S., Subramanian, S. K., Bhavanani, A. B., Sahai, A., & Thangavel, D. (2014). Effect of fast and slow pranayama practice on cognitive functions in healthy volunteers. Journal of clinical and diagnostic research: JCDR, 8(1), 10.

7. Telles, S., Yadav, A., Kumar, N., Sharma, S., Visweswaraiah, N. K., & Balkrishna, A. (2013). Blood pressure and Purdue pegboard scores in individuals with hypertension after alternate nostril breathing, breath awareness, and no intervention. Medical science monitor: international medical journal of experimental and clinical research, 19, 61.

8. Thanalakshmi, J., Maheshkumar, K., Kannan, R., Sundareswaran, L., Venugopal, V., & Poonguzhali, S. (2020). Effect of Sheetali pranayama on cardiac autonomic function among patients with primary hypertension-A randomized controlled trial. Complementary Therapies in Clinical Practice, 39, 101138.

9. Ubolnuar, N., Tantisuwat, A., Thaveeratitham, P., Lertmaharit, S., Kruapanich, C., & Mathiyakom, W. (2019). Effects of breathing exercises in patients with chronic obstructive pulmonary disease: systematic review and meta-analysis. Annals of rehabilitation medicine, 43(4), 509-523.

10. Ubolsakka-Jones, C., Sangthong, B., Khrisanapant, W., & Jones, D. A. (2017). The effect of slow-loaded breathing training on the blood pressure response to handgrip exercise in patients with isolated systolic hypertension. Hypertension Research, 40(10), 885-891.

11. Ubolsakka-Jones, C., Tongdee, P., & Jones, D. A. (2019). The effects of slow loaded breathing training on exercise blood pressure in isolated systolic hypertension. Physiotherapy Research International, 24(4), e1785.

12. Ublosakka-Jones, C., Tongdee, P., Pachirat, O., & Jones, D. A. (2018). Slow loaded breathing training improves blood pressure, lung capacity and arm exercise endurance for older people with treated and stable isolated systolic hypertension. Experimental Gerontology, 108, 48-53.

3.5 Marital status

Mc Causland et al. (2014) conducted an intriguing analysis, which, despite the fact that it was not an intervention, could be of interest to the readers. To be more specific, a study was conducted on a sample of American citizens to investigate the connection between married status and blood pressure. It was discovered that married people have statistically considerably lower blood pressure than single persons, with men experiencing a drop in blood pressure of 3.1 mm Hg and women experiencing a drop in blood pressure of 1.7 mm Hg. Furthermore, there was a distinction between married non-blacks and married blacks (-2.7 and -2.4 mm Hg, respectively).

References

1. Mc Causland, F. R., Sacks, F. M., & Forman, J. P. (2014). Marital status, dipping and nocturnal blood pressure: results from the Dietary Approaches to Stop Hypertension trial. Journal of hypertension, 32(4), 756-761.

3.6 Sauna

The effect that saunas have on blood pressure has only been investigated in a single study that was carried out by Gayda et al. (2012). Furthermore, the research focused on individual sessions, meaning that one of the sessions consisted solely of participants remaining in the sauna, while the other session combined sauna time with physical activity. Both of the quick interventions brought about a modest decrease in blood pressure and the difference was no more than 5 mm Hg.

References

1. Gayda, M., Paillard, F., Sosner, P., Juneau, M., Garzon, M., Gonzalez, M., ... & Nigam, A. (2012). Effects of sauna alone and postexercise sauna baths on blood pressure and hemodynamic variables in patients with untreated hypertension. The Journal of Clinical Hypertension, 14(8), 553-560.

3.7 Social media education

Despite the fact that the intervention that was described by Mancheno et al. (2021) did not result in a reduction in blood pressure, I thought it would be worthwhile to briefly discuss it owing to the nature of the intervention. The authors of the paper invited people who participated in a study with hypertension that was inadequately controlled to tweet or retweet items related to health twice per week for a period of six months. Participants' blood pressure was not shown to be reduced in any way, despite the fact that they were exposed to content relating to health.

References

1. Mancheno, C., Asch, D. A., Klinger, E. V., Goldshear, J. L., Mitra, N., Buttenheim, A. M., ... & Merchant, R. M. (2021). Effect of Posting on Social Media on Systolic Blood Pressure and Management of Hypertension: A Randomized Controlled Trial. Journal of the American Heart Association, 10(19), e020596.

3.8 Stress management

Two research studies reported the participants' engagement in stress-reduction activities (Blom et al. 2014, Clemow et al. 2018). The eight-week mindfulness-based stress reduction (MBSR) program that was employed in the study by Blom et al. (2014) did not result in a drop in the participants' blood pressure. On the other hand, the 10-week intervention led to a drop in blood pressure that was an average of 7.5 mm Hg lower in the second publication.

Stress management - how was the intervention conducted?

Clemow et al. (2018) discuss the implementation of a stress management program at the workplace in the form of group workshops that ran for a total of ten weeks and were carried out with workers with hypertension who were employed at urban medical centers. Participants attended ten meetings every week, each of which lasted for an hour. These sessions, which were led by experts in the field, took place at noon time on weekdays during the lunch period. These workshops, which were called LifeSkills, comprised a cognitive-behavioral group intervention. The program was based on cognitive-behavioral techniques and methods for stress reduction. The following topics were discussed and worked on throughout the session:

- identification and evaluation of thoughts, feelings and behaviors in response to stressful situations,
- problem solving,

- assertiveness in dealing with events and / or demands that cause anger and stress,
- deflexion skills to reduce distress in stressful situations, such as breathing and muscle relaxation, distraction and increasing stress tolerance
- ability to communicate,
- increasing empathy and building positive relationships.

These sessions also included the presentation of video materials that were connected to the theme.

This intervention resulted in a reduction of emotional exhaustion and depressive rumination, both of which correlated with a decrease in blood pressure, which was found to be 7.5 mm Hg lower on average.

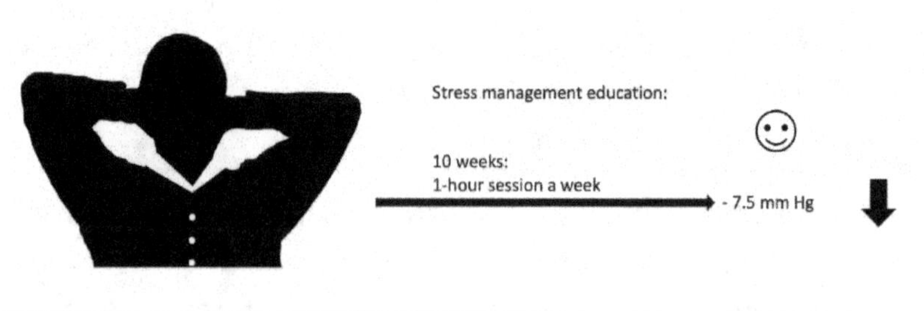

What you should know

- Minimizing daily stress is vital for one's health. This is due to the fact that prolonged exposure to stress is detrimental to one's health and raises the likelihood of developing illnesses such as coronary heart disease, anxiety disorders, and depression (Gallo et al. 2014).
- Participating in aerobic exercise twice per week was found to considerably lower stress in a trial that lasted for a period of six weeks (Herbert et al. 2020).
- According to a number of studies, those who have a diet that is heavy in ultra-processed foods as well as added sugar are

more likely to report feeling higher levels of perceived stress (Schweren et al. 2021).

- Both adults and children who spend an inordinate amount of time in front of screens have been found to have lower levels of psychological well-being and higher levels of stress as a result of this behavior (Twenge and Campbell 2018).

- Too much caffeine can make anxiety worse and make it harder to deal with. It's best to stay under 400 mg of caffeine per day, which is about 4–5 cups (0.9–1.2 L) of coffee (Evans and Griffiths 1999).

References

1. Blom, K., Baker, B., How, M., Dai, M., Irvine, J., Abbey, S., ... & Tobe, S. W. (2014). Hypertension analysis of stress reduction using mindfulness meditation and yoga: results from the harmony randomized controlled trial. American journal of Hypertension, 27(1), 122-129.
2. Clemow, L. P., Pickering, T. G., Davidson, K. W., Schwartz, J. E., Williams, V. P., Shaffer, J. A., ... & Gerin, W. (2018). Stress management in the workplace for employees with hypertension: a randomized controlled trial. Translational behavioral medicine, 8(5), 761-770.
3. Evans, S. M., & Griffiths, R. R. (1999). Caffeine withdrawal: a parametric analysis of caffeine dosing conditions. Journal of Pharmacology and Experimental Therapeutics, 289(1), 285-294.
4. Gallo, L. C., Roesch, S. C., Fortmann, A. L., Carnethon, M. R., Penedo, F. J., Perreira, K., ... & Isasi, C. R. (2014). Associations of chronic stress burden, perceived stress, and traumatic stress with cardiovascular disease prevalence and risk factors in the HCHS/SOL Sociocultural Ancillary Study. Psychosomatic medicine, 76(6), 468.
5. Herbert, C., Meixner, F., Wiebking, C., & Gilg, V. (2020). Regular physical activity, short-term exercise, mental health, and well-being among university students: the results of an online and a laboratory study. Frontiers in psychology, 11, 509.
6. Schweren, L. J., Larsson, H., Vinke, P. C., Li, L., Kvalvik, L. G., Arias-Vasquez, A., ... & Hartman, C. A. (2021). Diet quality, stress and common mental health problems: A cohort study of 121,008 adults. Clinical Nutrition, 40(3), 901-906.
7. Twenge, J. M., & Campbell, W. K. (2018). Associations between screen time and lower psychological well-being among children and adolescents: Evidence from a population-based study. Preventive medicine reports, 12, 271-283.

3.9 Yoga

Seven studies have been done in the last 10 years to find out if yoga can lower blood pressure. Surprisingly, there was no statistically significant effect in three publications (Hagins et al. 2014, Wolff et al. 2013, 2016). Furthermore, in another three publications (Cramer et al. 2018, Dhameja et al. 2013, Roche et al. 2017), the effect was not very large, i.e., a blood pressure reduction of 2.56-3.8 mm Hg was reported. Only a single study of Roche et al. (2017) yielded noticeable results.

Yoga - how was the intervention conducted?

The study, which was conducted by Roche et al. (2017), lasted for a period of three months and required participants to attend a total of twenty-six yoga sessions. All of the participants were locals of the island of Gran Canaria and ranged in age from 40 to 71. Each of the sessions lasted for one hour and ninety minutes, and they occurred twice per week. It is known that the program of yoga techniques was based on the practice of postures (asanas) and breathing techniques that are expressly advised for the treatment of hypertension. However, the authors of the publication do not say exactly what techniques were applied in the study. In addition to meditation and other practices of attention and awareness, yogic relaxation and visualization techniques were also incorporated. The intervention led to a decrease in blood pressure among the participants of 12.4 mm Hg, on average.

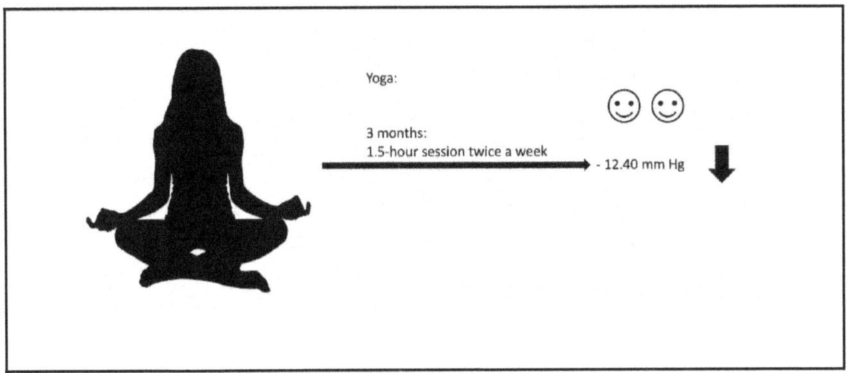

What you should know

- The results indicate that 6 weeks of single-session yoga training (one 90-minute session per week) may be useful for enhancing the flexibility of the erector spinae and hamstrings (Amin and Goodman 2014).

- There is some evidence which suggests that yoga can be helpful in lowering levels of stress, anxiety, and depression (Shohani et al. 2018).

- Yoga has been shown to be an effective method for lowering inflammatory responses in a wide variety of chronic illnesses (Djalilova et al. 2019).

- According to the findings of one study, practicing yoga for only twelve minutes every day can considerably enhance bone health (Lu et al. 2016).

References

1. Amin, D. J., & Goodman, M. (2014). The effects of selected asanas in Iyengar yoga on flexibility: Pilot study. Journal of bodywork and movement therapies, 18(3), 399-404.
2. Cramer, H., Sellin, C., Schumann, D., & Dobos, G. (2018). Yoga in arterial hypertension: A three-armed, randomized controlled trial. Deutsches Ärzteblatt International, 115(50), 833.
3. Dhameja, K., Singh, S., Mustafa, M. D., Singh, K. P., Banerjee, B. D., Agarwal, M., & Ahmed, R. S. (2013). Therapeutic effect of yoga in patients with hypertension with reference to GST gene polymorphism. The Journal of Alternative and Complementary Medicine, 19(3), 243-249.

4. Djalilova, D. M., Schulz, P. S., Berger, A. M., Case, A. J., Kupzyk, K. A., & Ross, A. C. (2019). Impact of yoga on inflammatory biomarkers: a systematic review. Biological research for nursing, 21(2), 198-209.

5. Hagins, M., Rundle, A., Consedine, N. S., & Khalsa, S. B. S. (2014). A randomized controlled trial comparing the effects of yoga with an active control on ambulatory blood pressure in individuals with prehypertension and stage 1 hypertension. The Journal of Clinical Hypertension, 16(1), 54-62.

6. Lu, Y. H., Rosner, B., Chang, G., & Fishman, L. M. (2016). Twelve-minute daily yoga regimen reverses osteoporotic bone loss. Topics in geriatric rehabilitation, 32(2), 81.

7. Roche, L. T., Barrachina, M. T. M., Fernández, I. I., & Betancort, M. (2017). YOGA and self-regulation in management of essential arterial hypertension and associated emotional symptomatology: A randomized controlled trial.

8. Shohani, M., Badfar, G., Nasirkandy, M. P., Kaikhavani, S., Rahmati, S., Modmeli, Y., ... & Azami, M. (2018). The effect of yoga on stress, anxiety, and depression in women. International journal of preventive medicine, 9.

9. Wolff, M., Rogers, K., Erdal, B., Chalmers, J. P., Sundquist, K., & Midlöv, P. (2016). Impact of a short home-based yoga programme on blood pressure in patients with hypertension: a randomized controlled trial in primary care. Journal of human hypertension, 30(10), 599-605.

10. Wolff, M., Sundquist, K., Larsson Lönn, S., & Midlöv, P. (2013). Impact of yoga on blood pressure and quality of life in patients with hypertension–a controlled trial in primary care, matched for systolic blood pressure. BMC cardiovascular disorders, 13(1), 1-9.

3.10 Summary of other interventions - what works?

In this chapter, the impacts of factors that are not classified anywhere else in this book were examined. The highest number of publications that did not show an association between the chosen intervention and blood pressure concerned yoga (three out of seven total), followed by breathing training (two out of nine total), and finally, acupressure, acupuncture, behavioral or lifestyle modifications, social media education, and stress management, each receiving one publication with non-significant statistical results.

Publications on breathing training (five of which showed an average blood pressure decrease of at least 13.38 mm Hg), as well as behavioral and lifestyle modifications (4 experiments achieved a reduction of more than 10 mm Hg on average), were shown to have the biggest average reduction in blood pressure.

It is important to note that interventions such as acupressure, acupuncture, and yoga have not demonstrated much of an effect on blood pressure, and the results have also frequently been inconclusive.

PART 4. SUMMARY OF ALL DESCRIBED INTERVENTIONS

The book discusses over fifty distinct interventions that have had varying degrees of impact on blood pressure. Of course, these are not all of the research studies that have been conducted on the subject; I acknowledged that at the beginning. As I needed to cut down on the amount of information I would need to compile for this book, I made the decision to focus on the most recent decade and take into account the results of all clinical studies on hypertension that have been published in the PubMed database during that time period. I believe that this is enough material to consider that the data paints a positive image of those groups of interventions that have a chance of actually lowering blood pressure. Of course, I recommend not treating all this as the Holy Grail, although these are certainly valuable tips on how to change your diet or lifestyle in general to support the treatment of hypertension or even prevent its development. What is very important - I do not recommend that you follow the mentioned methodologies without consulting a medically trained specialist. And most importantly never, ever, ever, abandon the therapies recommended by medical experts in favor of the methods listed here, unless, for example, your doctor suggests such a change. I recommend special caution with supplements (especially herbs), which can interact with drugs by strengthening or weakening their effects.

In the section on dietary interventions (1.1), the most effective intervention was the DASH diet adjusted by adaptation to the Japanese diet (blood pressure lowered by 16.94-23 mm Hg), or paired with physical activity (blood pressure reduced by 16.1-17.6 mm Hg), or significantly reduced salt intake (reduced by 14.4-17 mm Hg). Consumption of oat bran was also associated with successful outcomes (reduced by 15.3 mm Hg).

The supplementation described in section 1.2 demonstrated that the most effective interventions for high blood pressure included the use of Indian kudzu (which lowered blood pressure by 25 mm Hg), Mellisa officinalis (which lowered blood pressure by 21.45 mm Hg), quercetin (which reduced blood pressure by 19.5 mm Hg), American ginseng (which reduced blood pressure by 17.4 mm Hg), and Orthosiphon stamineus (blood pressure decreased by 15 mm Hg). Supplementation with flaxseed, Fufang Danshen, and African traditional medicines all led to reductions in blood pressure that were greater than or equivalent to 10 mm Hg. Once again, I will remind you that I do not recommend supplementation without consulting a medical professional.

In the section of the book dedicated to physical activity (sections 2.1, 2.2, and 2.3), it is made abundantly clear that aerobic training is superior than anaerobic training in terms of results connected with blood pressure reduction. Of course, these conclusions are in line with generally accepted guidelines, although the devil is in the detail. The most effective interventions in all physical activity looking at the highest achieved reductions in hypertension were found to be training sessions in a heated pool, qigong (che-gong) classes (combines aerobic, isometric, and isotonic elements with meditation and relaxation) and interval training.

In other articles (part 3), breathing training and the outcomes gained through the application of behavioral or lifestyle change deserve special note. These results include a drop in blood pressure of up to 17-18 mm Hg.

I made a visualization, in which I incorporated only the most favorable of the results I found (Figure 8). This prevents the suppression of interventions that have only undergone a single trial within the past ten years (please see the analysis I elaborated on further down). It is important to point out that as a consequence of this summary, it might be simpler to contest it. Despite this, it does not imply that these findings should not be taken into consideration in any way. It's possible that they will work well for certain individuals (just as they came out in the studies).

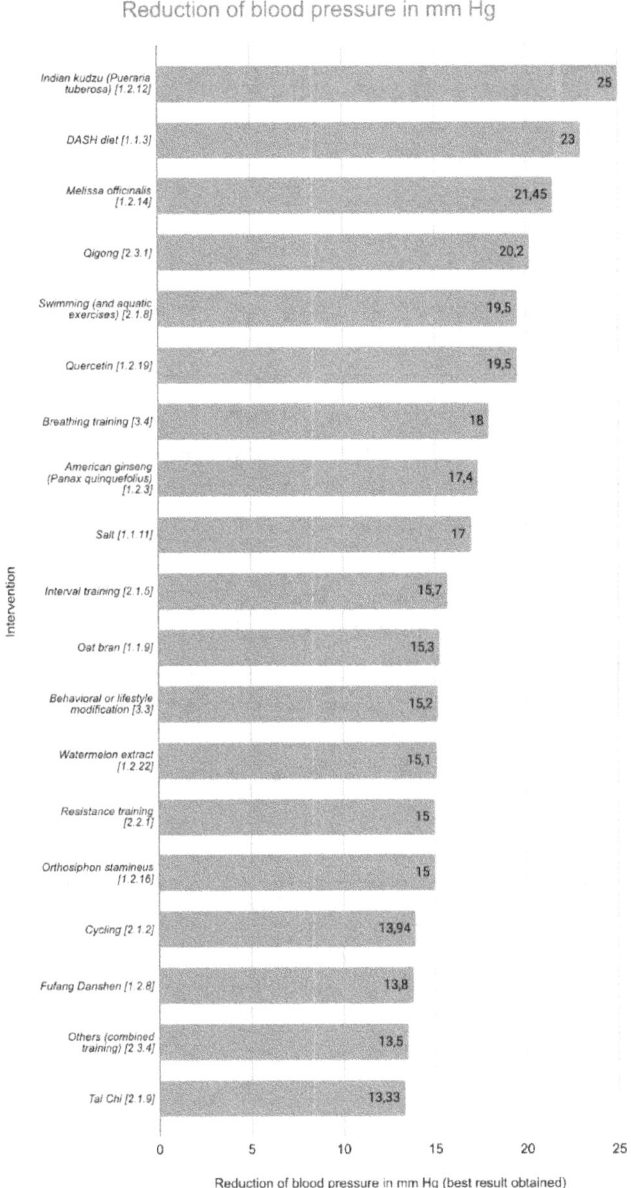

Figure 8. Comparison of all interventions described in this book based on a comparison of the best results obtained. Many of the interventions are described in single publications and therefore should be interpreted with caution.

The types of interventions that have been determined to be the most effective based on the highest levels of blood pressure reduction that researchers have attained are mentioned above. On the other hand, it makes a great deal of sense to take into account all of the findings that have been acquired in a specific field. To do this for the purposes of this book, I developed a fairly simple methodology that awards a given intervention 1 point for achieving a blood pressure reduction of more than 15 mm Hg, 0.5 points for a blood pressure reduction in subjects between 7 and 15 mm Hg, 0.25 points for a blood pressure reduction between more than 0 and up to 7 mm Hg (but a statistically significant blood pressure reduction is shown). On the other hand, where no statistically significant result was shown, I subtracted 0.75 points from the sum of all interventions in a given category for each such publication. In these calculations, I have disregarded one-time interventions because, despite the fact that I have discussed them in earlier sections, I felt it was inappropriate to compare them with methodologies that were implemented over the course of several weeks or months. According to this methodology, the type of intervention with the highest score was awarded 5 points; therefore, in order to better visualize this data, I changed it to a scale from 1-10 by multiplying each score by 2. The findings of this investigation are depicted in Figure 9 below. This calculation technique gives an advantage to those different sorts of interventions that are described in a greater number of publications, and therefore also those that have received more attention from researchers.

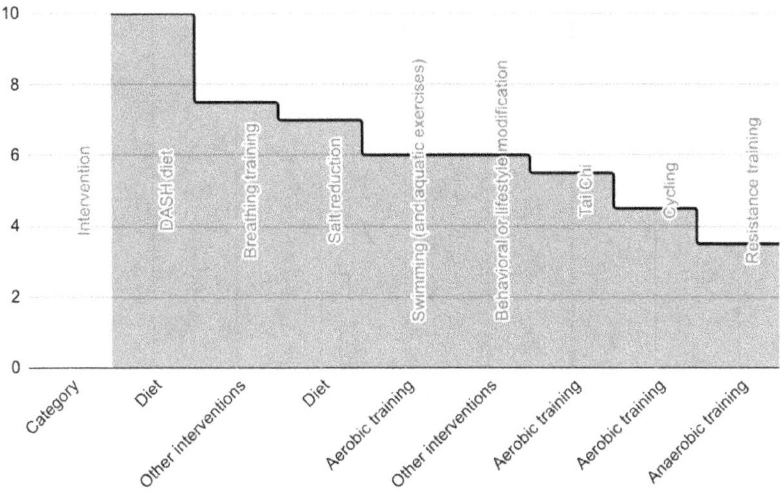

Figure 9. Interventions that have shown the highest impact on blood pressure. Interventions represented by a larger number of publications are given preference in this methodology.

Where can you find these methodologies?

- DASH diet - 1.1.3
- Breathing training - 3.4
- Salt reduction - 1.1.11
- Swimming (and aquatic exercises) - 2.1.8
- Behavioral or lifestyle modification - 3.3
- Tai Chi - 2.1.9
- Cycling - 2.1.2
- Resistance training - 2.2.1

In conclusion, it is challenging to declare with total conviction which of the two analyses presented in Figures 8 and 9 is the more accurate. Given the whole picture, I would probably recommend first paying attention to the interventions shown in Figure 9 as those that have been tested far more often and on different groups of participants. Although the interventions depicted in Figure 8 frequently demonstrated high efficacy, this effect is limited by the fact that they were typically carried out in single investigations.

ABOUT THE AUTHOR

I have a background in biotechnology and hold degrees in the biological sciences. So far in my career, I have been employed at several universities in Poland. In addition, I have participated in a number of research and development projects, many of which I have initiated and led. I am the author or co-author of dozens of scientific and popular science publications and more than a dozen biotechnology patents. I have experience managing both biotechnology enterprises and the scientific sections of companies that focus on developing novel biotechnologies. It is one of my greatest passions to enlighten people about the wonders of science, both in terms of what we already know and what the future may hold. I appreciate studying, and I love challenges.